Polymyalgia Rheumatica Quackery

Exposing Myths and Dangerous Treatments

Cheryl White MAT

Dr. Shane Wilson.

Copyright © 2024 Cheryl White, Shane Wilson

All rights reserved.

ISBN: 9798344454306

Contents

Contents	iii
1 Introduction	1
2 The Evolution of Quackery	7
3 A Dangerous Misalignment	13
4 Cranial Therapy: Risks and Realities	19
5 PMR Diet Myths and Facts	25
6 Other Pseudoscientific Diets	31
7 Diluting Reality	37
8 Energy Healing: Promises Without Proof	45
9 Flushing Out False Hopes	51
10 Misleading Nature's Potential	57
11 Uncredible Aromatherapy	63
12 Needles and Nonsense	69
13 A Breath of False Hope	75
14 How to Research on Your Own	81
15 Proven Treatments for PMR	87
17 FAQ	93
17 Conclusion	99
About the Authors	105

1 Introduction

When faced with a chronic illness like Polymyalgia Rheumatica (PMR), the journey toward relief often involves exploring a variety of treatment options. PMR is a complex, inflammatory condition that affects adults over the age of 50, causing pain, stiffness, and tenderness, especially in the shoulders, hips, and neck. Typically, PMR symptoms worsen in the morning and can significantly impair daily function, making even simple tasks feel challenging. Although the cause of PMR remains unknown, it is believed to be an autoimmune disorder, where the immune system mistakenly attacks the body's own tissues, resulting in inflammation.

The standard medical treatment for PMR usually includes low doses of corticosteroids like prednisone, which are effective in managing inflammation and reducing symptoms. Most patients experience improvement within days of starting corticosteroid therapy, which confirms the effectiveness of this approach. However, corticosteroids are often needed for prolonged periods to keep PMR symptoms in check. Unfortunately, long-term corticosteroid use brings risks, including weight gain, increased blood pressure, mood changes, osteoporosis, and elevated blood sugar. Some patients may also be prescribed additional medications like methotrexate to reduce their dependence on steroids and manage inflammation.

For many patients, the side effects and lifelong nature of treatment drive them to explore non-traditional or "natural" alternatives, especially when presented with the overwhelming landscape of online health advice. The internet is filled with self-styled health experts and unverified alternative medicine options promising "natural" cures or treatments for PMR. While some treatments may sound promising, many lack scientific backing and can lead patients down a potentially harmful path. This book, *Polymyalgia Rheumatica Quackery*, seeks to provide patients, families, and healthcare professionals with the knowledge and tools to critically evaluate the information surrounding PMR. By understanding which treatments are legitimate and which are fraudulent, patients can make informed decisions about managing their condition.

Why Quackery Thrives: The Draw of Alternative Treatments

Before diving into specific alternative treatments, it is important to understand why quackery—unscientific and fraudulent health practices—continues to attract patients. The history of quackery is as old as medicine itself; before the scientific era, people relied on folk remedies and charismatic healers to find solutions for ailments. Although scientific advancements have led to effective treatments for many conditions, the internet has also fueled the growth of modern-day quackery by giving everyone a platform.

Many factors draw people toward alternative treatments for conditions like PMR:

1. **Fear of Long-Term Medication:** Corticosteroids, though effective, carry risks when used long-term. Patients often look for "natural" options that promise similar relief without side effects, making them vulnerable to treatments that exploit these fears.

2. **Frustration with Medical Complexity:** PMR is challenging to diagnose and manage. Symptoms may fluctuate, and improvement can feel slow. In response, patients may turn to alternative treatments that provide overly simplistic explanations for their problems.

3. **Desire for Control:** Living with PMR can make patients feel powerless, especially when dependent on medication. Alternative treatments often provide an illusion of control, leading patients to believe they can manage their symptoms through lifestyle changes alone.

4. **Emotional Vulnerability:** PMR's chronic pain and fatigue can leave patients feeling desperate for a cure. Quack practitioners often exploit this desperation, offering "miracle cures" to those willing to try anything for relief.

5. **Pervasive Misinformation:** The internet makes it difficult to distinguish credible medical advice from pseudoscience. Professional-looking websites and personal testimonials give legitimacy to treatments that lack scientific support.

Understanding Polymyalgia Rheumatica

PMR is one of the most common inflammatory disorders in older adults, yet its cause remains unknown. It is characterized by symptoms such as stiffness, pain, and tenderness in areas like the shoulders, hips, and neck. These symptoms often appear suddenly, without any prior indication of illness, and are typically most severe in the morning. While PMR is manageable with treatment, it often requires a long-term commitment to corticosteroids, which come with side effects. This dependence on medication can be daunting, leading patients to seek alternative or supplementary treatments. However, it is important to understand that PMR cannot be cured through diet or detoxification alone; it is a systemic condition that requires targeted treatment to control inflammation and prevent complications.

Debunking Common Alternative Treatments for PMR

As patients search for relief, they may encounter various popular but unproven "cures" for PMR. Below are some of the most common forms of quackery and the reasons why they are ineffective or even harmful.

Diet-Based Cures: Separating Fact from Fiction

One of the most prevalent myths in alternative PMR treatment is the belief that specific diets can cure or reverse the condition. Among the popular recommendations are the anti-inflammatory, vegan, and alkaline diets, all of which claim to reduce inflammation, detoxify the body, or "balance" internal pH levels.

While eating a balanced diet rich in fruits, vegetables, and whole grains can support overall health, there is no evidence that it can replace corticosteroids for managing PMR. The anti-inflammatory diet, which includes omega-3 fatty acids and antioxidants, may alleviate some general inflammation in the body, but it cannot directly address the autoimmune response that drives PMR. Similarly, vegan and alkaline diets, despite claims of detoxification and pH balance, lack scientific support for influencing the body's immune response.

Detoxification and Supplement Myths

The concept of "detoxifying" the body through cleanses, fasting, or supplements is popular in alternative medicine. Many PMR patients are advised to "reset" their systems through restrictive diets or supplements that claim to remove toxins and reduce inflammation. These treatments often involve drinking specific juices, fasting, or consuming expensive supplements.

However, the body is naturally equipped with efficient detoxification systems—the liver and kidneys handle this task well without external help. There is no scientific evidence that detox programs can influence PMR symptoms or that the body accumulates toxins that contribute to this condition. Supplements like fish oil and turmeric, while offering mild anti-inflammatory properties, are not substitutes for prescribed medications. In some cases, supplements can interfere with medications, leading to unintended side effects.

The Illusion of Energy Healing and Reiki

Energy healing practices, such as Reiki, claim to channel energy to restore balance and promote healing. Practitioners suggest that these therapies can alleviate PMR symptoms by "rebalancing" the body's energy. While such practices may offer relaxation and comfort to some, there is no scientific evidence that energy healing can impact PMR or alter the autoimmune mechanisms underlying it. Relying on energy healing in place of proven treatments risks delaying necessary medical intervention, which can worsen symptoms over time.

Pseudoscience and the Influence of Online Communities

One of the most concerning trends in alternative treatments is the role of online communities that perpetuate misinformation. Social media, blogs, and YouTube channels dedicated to alternative PMR treatments create echo chambers, reinforcing beliefs that quack remedies work and that conventional medicine is harmful.

Such communities often thrive on anecdotal testimonials and conspiracy theories that suggest the medical community is withholding cures. Patients, often isolated and in search of support, may feel validated by these communities, even though the treatments promoted lack scientific grounding.

The Importance of Evidence-Based Medicine and Critical Thinking

PMR requires careful management under the supervision of qualified medical professionals. Though alternative treatments may seem appealing, patients should approach any treatment with a healthy dose of skepticism and prioritize evidence-based options. Critical thinking, particularly in the face of persuasive online claims, is essential to avoid the risks associated with unproven treatments.

Here are some general tips for evaluating PMR treatments:

1. **Question Miracle Cures:** No legitimate treatment offers an immediate cure for PMR. Be wary of any approach that promises rapid results without the use of conventional medicine.

2. **Evaluate Sources:** Focus on credible sources like peer-

reviewed journals, established health organizations, and licensed medical professionals.

3. **Seek Professional Guidance:** Open communication with healthcare providers can help patients explore their options safely. Medical professionals can provide insights into the effectiveness of different treatments and explain why certain methods, like corticosteroids, remain the standard.

4. **Watch for Pseudoscience Clues:** Treatments that rely on anecdotal evidence, use terms like "toxin buildup," or focus on broad, undefined benefits are likely pseudoscientific.

Conclusion: A Path Toward Safe and Effective PMR Management

Polymyalgia Rheumatica is a complex and challenging condition that requires appropriate medical care for effective management. Although it is natural to seek alternatives when faced with the burdens of chronic illness, quack treatments that claim to cure or replace conventional medicine can be harmful. By equipping yourself with the tools of critical thinking and understanding the legitimate science behind PMR, you can make informed choices that prioritize safety and well-being.

As you navigate your PMR journey, remember that managing this condition is a gradual process that involves balancing the benefits and risks of all treatments. Evidence-based medicine provides a pathway to symptom control, but it may take time to achieve the best possible outcome. By focusing on reliable treatments and maintaining open conversations with healthcare providers, you empower yourself to take control of your health and well-being.

2 The Evolution of Quackery

Quackery is a longstanding practice involving the promotion and sale of unproven, often dangerous medical treatments. A "quack" is someone who falsely claims medical expertise or sells remedies that promise to cure without scientific evidence. Throughout history, quackery has taken various forms, from "miracle" elixirs to bizarre surgeries, and it has attracted countless individuals desperate for relief from their ailments. For those with conditions like Polymyalgia Rheumatica (PMR), where the pain and limited options can feel overwhelming, the temptation of alternative treatments is often heightened. Understanding the history of quackery provides context for why these treatments appeal to patients today and highlights the need for vigilance to protect vulnerable individuals from potentially harmful choices.

The term "quack" derives from the Dutch word "quacksalver," meaning "hawker of salves" or "peddler of ointments." During the Middle Ages, "quacksalvers" were street vendors who loudly promoted homemade remedies, claiming miraculous benefits in public markets and squares. Known for their charisma and flair, these individuals attracted large crowds by promising quick cures for various ailments. Over time, "quack" became synonymous with medical fraud, as these peddlers often lacked any real medical knowledge, selling treatments that were either ineffective or dangerous.

Historically, quacks thrived during times when medical knowledge was limited and access to legitimate medical care was scarce. Before modern science, people relied on folk remedies, superstitions, and persuasive healers to manage their illnesses. Quacks exploited the fear and desperation of those suffering from chronic or incurable illnesses, offering "cures" when conventional medicine had little to offer. Despite advancements in science and medicine, quackery has evolved to suit modern concerns, adapting its tactics to fit emerging diseases and chronic conditions, including PMR.

Notorious Quack Remedies in History

Some of the most infamous quack treatments in history gained widespread acceptance before their harmful effects were discovered. Here are some notorious examples that illustrate the lengths to which quackery has gone, often with devastating consequences:

1. **Radium Water**
   In the early 20th century, radium, a radioactive element, was marketed as a miracle cure for a range of ailments, from arthritis to impotence. "Radium water" was sold as a tonic believed to "recharge" the body with energy. Tragically, it caused severe radiation poisoning, leading to horrific injuries and deaths. One of the most famous cases was that of Eben Byers, a wealthy industrialist who consumed large quantities of radium water, eventually dying a painful death as parts of his jaw deteriorated due to radiation poisoning.

2. **Bloodletting**
   Bloodletting was widely practiced for centuries to treat ailments as diverse as infections, fevers, and mental illness. Based on the ancient theory of balancing bodily "humors," physicians believed that draining blood would restore health. This practice persisted for hundreds of years, often weakening patients further or leading to death from blood

loss. While based on a flawed understanding of human physiology, bloodletting demonstrates how deeply embedded quackery can become in the medical community.

3. **Snake Oil**
"Snake oil" originally referred to oils derived from the Chinese water snake, which has some anti-inflammatory properties. However, in 19th-century America, traveling salesmen began selling fake snake oil remedies, often containing little more than mineral oil or turpentine. These dubious products were marketed as cures for arthritis, pain, and inflammation, giving rise to the modern metaphor for fraudulent health products.

4. **Mercury and Arsenic Cures**
In the 18th and 19th centuries, mercury and arsenic were commonly used in medicines, particularly for syphilis and tuberculosis. These toxic elements caused severe side effects, including hair loss, neurological damage, and death. Despite the evident dangers, these "remedies" were accepted due to the lack of effective treatments for certain diseases.

5. **Dr. John Brinkley's Goat Gland Surgery**
In the 1920s, Dr. John Brinkley claimed he could cure male impotence by implanting goat testicles into men. Despite having no formal medical training, he became wealthy and famous, performing thousands of surgeries. His methods led to numerous deaths, complications, and lawsuits, and eventually, his medical license was revoked. Brinkley's case is one of the most bizarre and extreme examples of medical quackery.

Why Quackery Appeals to PMR Patients

Polymyalgia Rheumatica (PMR) is a chronic inflammatory condition that causes severe pain and stiffness, especially in the shoulders and hips. The standard treatment is corticosteroids, which are generally effective in managing symptoms. However, long-term steroid use brings potential side effects, including weight gain, high blood pressure, mood changes, and bone density loss. These side effects, along with the unpredictability of PMR symptoms and lack of a definitive cure, make some patients more susceptible to alternative or "miracle" treatments.

Driving PMR Patients Toward Quack Treatments

1. **Chronic Pain and Stiffness**
   PMR patients deal with ongoing pain and stiffness that makes even simple tasks challenging. When conventional treatments fall short, patients may feel desperate to try anything for relief. Quack treatments often promise quick fixes, appealing to this need for relief.

2. **Fear of Long-Term Medication Side Effects**
   Corticosteroids are a standard treatment for PMR but come with side effects that can be hard to manage. Patients may feel that exploring "natural" treatments is a safer option. Quack treatments often exploit this fear, advertising unverified supplements or therapies as safer alternatives.

3. **Frustration with Flare-Ups**
   PMR symptoms can vary, with periods of remission followed by flare-ups. This unpredictability can be frustrating, and quacks may claim that their treatments can prevent flare-ups or eliminate inflammation, offering patients a false sense of control.

4. **Lack of Awareness and Support**
   PMR, though common in older adults, is not widely understood. Patients may feel isolated or struggle to find doctors familiar with their condition. The lack of support can drive some patients to seek alternative therapies from individuals who claim to understand their symptoms and offer empathy, even if they lack legitimate solutions.

5. **Online Misinformation and Pseudoscience**
   The internet is filled with pseudoscientific health advice. YouTube videos, forums, and social media accounts

promote "natural cures" for PMR that lack any scientific support. Patients are vulnerable to these messages, especially when feeling desperate for answers.

Dangerous Quack Treatments for PMR

Modern quack treatments can be risky for PMR patients, not only because they are ineffective but also because they can delay proper care and interact dangerously with prescribed medications.

- **Unregulated Supplements**: Many quack practitioners recommend supplements to reduce inflammation or "boost immunity." Supplements are not regulated by the FDA, meaning their effectiveness and safety are not verified. Certain supplements may interfere with medications, causing adverse effects.

- **Detox Programs**: Detox programs promise to "cleanse" the body of toxins, often requiring fasting, restrictive diets, or herbal supplements. However, the body's liver and kidneys naturally detoxify, and detox programs offer no benefits for autoimmune conditions like PMR. They can lead to dehydration, malnutrition, and other health risks.

- **Energy Healing and Reiki**: Practices like Reiki, which claim to channel energy for healing, may provide temporary relaxation, but there's no scientific basis for using them to treat PMR. While such therapies might offer a placebo effect, relying on them instead of proven treatments can allow symptoms to worsen.

- **Miracle Diets and Fads**: Diet-based quack treatments, such as the alkaline diet, anti-inflammatory diet, and gluten-free diet, are often marketed as cures for autoimmune conditions. While a balanced diet can promote general health, these diets lack evidence for managing or curing PMR. Restrictive diets may lead to nutritional deficiencies without addressing the condition's root cause.

The Importance of Evidence-Based Medicine

Quack treatments pose real risks to PMR patients, who require evidence-based treatments to manage their symptoms safely. Staying informed and critically evaluating health information is essential to avoid falling prey to pseudoscientific claims. Patients can use the following strategies to protect themselves:

1. **Question Miracle Cures**: Any treatment that claims to cure PMR quickly and without conventional medicine is likely a scam.

2. **Seek Reputable Sources**: Consult peer-reviewed journals, respected health organizations, and licensed medical professionals for advice on managing PMR.

3. **Communicate with Healthcare Providers**: Patients may feel hesitant to discuss alternative treatments with their doctors, but open dialogue can provide valuable insights into why certain treatments work and others don't.

4. **Watch for Red Flags**: Be wary of treatments that rely on anecdotal evidence, use phrases like "toxin buildup," or promise benefits beyond what science supports.

In conclusion, quackery has existed throughout history, exploiting the vulnerable in the name of profit. For patients with PMR, a complex and often debilitating condition, the allure of quick fixes and miracle cures is understandable but dangerous. By understanding the history of quackery and recognizing its modern manifestations, patients can protect themselves from false hope and potentially harmful treatments.

3 A Dangerous Misalignment

Chiropractic treatment is a popular alternative therapy often used to treat musculoskeletal problems like back pain, neck pain, and joint stiffness. Chiropractors, who focus on the alignment of the spine, believe that spinal adjustments can relieve pressure, restore mobility, and even treat a wide range of non-musculoskeletal conditions. However, when it comes to conditions like Polymyalgia Rheumatica (PMR)—a chronic inflammatory disorder causing widespread muscle pain and stiffness—chiropractic care enters dangerous territory. PMR affects the muscles rather than the spine directly, and the inflammation driving the disease process cannot be alleviated by spinal adjustments. Despite some chiropractors claiming they can relieve or cure PMR symptoms, there is no scientific evidence to support these claims. In fact, chiropractic manipulations can pose significant risks to PMR patients, sometimes worsening symptoms or causing unnecessary delays in receiving appropriate medical care. This chapter will explore the dangers of chiropractic care for PMR patients, provide patient stories as cautionary examples, and examine the controversies surrounding chiropractic adjustments.

Chiropractic Adjustments and PMR: A Mismatch in Treatment

Polymyalgia Rheumatica primarily affects muscles, particularly in the shoulders, hips, and neck, leading to pain and stiffness, especially in the morning or after periods of inactivity. The underlying cause of PMR is systemic inflammation, which is why treatment typically involves corticosteroids to reduce inflammation and improve quality of life. However, chiropractic adjustments focus on the spine and musculoskeletal alignment, a completely different approach to what PMR patients need. Any claim that chiropractic adjustments can alleviate or cure PMR is misleading at best and dangerous at worst.

Chiropractic care typically aims to relieve pressure on nerves and joints through spinal manipulations. While this may provide temporary relief for certain musculoskeletal problems, PMR requires treatment that addresses the immune system's inflammatory response, not the alignment of the spine. Chiropractic adjustments, particularly those involving aggressive manipulations, do nothing to address the root cause of PMR and may even exacerbate the pain and stiffness that patients experience. For instance, neck manipulations could worsen muscle pain or cause injury in already compromised or inflamed muscles. This makes chiropractic care an ineffective and risky option for those suffering from PMR.

Patient Stories: The Risks of Chiropractic Adjustments for PMR

Patient stories provide a stark warning of the potential dangers of chiropractic care for PMR. One example involved a 67-year-old woman diagnosed with PMR who sought chiropractic care after growing frustrated with the side effects of her prescribed corticosteroids. Her chiropractor assured her that regular spinal adjustments would help manage her pain. Over the course of several weeks, she underwent frequent manipulations, but instead of finding relief, she began experiencing worsening pain in her shoulders and hips. After a particularly intense session focusing on her neck and upper spine, she noticed increased stiffness and difficulty raising her arms.

Eventually, the woman's general practitioner ordered blood tests that showed elevated inflammatory markers consistent with PMR, confirming that the chiropractic care had done nothing to treat the underlying inflammation. Worse, the delay in returning to her prescribed corticosteroids allowed her symptoms to worsen significantly, prolonging her recovery.

Another cautionary tale comes from a 72-year-old man with PMR who was lured by a chiropractor's claims that spinal adjustments could help with his muscle pain. Although skeptical, the man was desperate to find an alternative to long-term steroid use. After several sessions, his stiffness and fatigue worsened, and he began to experience severe headaches—a side effect of the manipulations. A rheumatologist later explained that the manipulations had put additional stress on his already inflamed muscles, likely exacerbating his condition. The man was forced to return to a higher dose of corticosteroids to control the inflammation, a setback that could have been avoided with appropriate medical treatment from the start.

These stories demonstrate how chiropractic care can worsen PMR symptoms and cause unnecessary suffering. By relying on unproven treatments, patients often delay or avoid the medical care they need, allowing their condition to deteriorate and complicating their treatment plans in the long run.

The History and Controversies of Chiropractic Adjustments

The practice of chiropractic care was founded by Daniel David Palmer in the late 19th century. Palmer believed that misalignments of the spine, which he called "subluxations," were the root cause of many health problems. He theorized that by adjusting the spine, chiropractors could correct these subluxations and restore the body's natural ability to heal itself. While chiropractic care has gained mainstream acceptance for treating musculoskeletal issues like back pain, it remains controversial, particularly when applied to conditions like PMR, where systemic inflammation, not spinal misalignment, is the cause of pain.

One of the most contentious aspects of chiropractic care is the lack of scientific evidence supporting the chiropractic subluxation theory. Many chiropractors claim that spinal adjustments can treat a wide range of health problems, including inflammatory conditions like PMR. However, these claims are not supported by rigorous scientific research. Numerous studies have failed to demonstrate any measurable health benefits from chiropractic adjustments beyond temporary relief from musculoskeletal pain, and no evidence supports their use in treating autoimmune or inflammatory conditions like PMR.

In the case of PMR, the subluxation theory is irrelevant because the pain and stiffness patients experience are due to inflammation, not spinal misalignment. Chiropractors who claim they can treat PMR are engaging in medical misinformation, putting vulnerable patients at risk. This is particularly concerning because patients with PMR may be desperate to find alternatives to corticosteroids due to their side effects, making them more susceptible to false promises.

Finding a Good Chiropractor: Why It's Difficult for PMR Patients

For patients seeking chiropractic care, one of the biggest challenges is finding a reputable practitioner. The chiropractic industry is largely unregulated compared to other medical fields, and there is significant variation in the quality of care provided by chiropractors. Some chiropractors focus on evidence-based treatments for musculoskeletal issues, while others embrace the subluxation theory and claim to treat a wide range of unrelated health conditions, including inflammatory disorders like PMR.

This lack of regulation can be especially dangerous for PMR patients. Because PMR symptoms—such as pain and stiffness in the shoulders, neck, and hips—can resemble musculoskeletal problems, some chiropractors may believe they can treat these symptoms without understanding the underlying inflammatory cause. This can lead to inappropriate and harmful treatments, such as aggressive manipulations that worsen muscle pain and delay proper medical intervention.

Chiropractic Care vs. Medical Treatment for PMR: Why Medical Management Is Essential

For patients with Polymyalgia Rheumatica, proper medical care is essential. The standard treatment for PMR involves corticosteroids, which help reduce inflammation and relieve pain. This medical approach targets the root cause of PMR: the immune system's inflammatory response. While chiropractic adjustments may offer temporary relief for general musculoskeletal pain, they are not a substitute for medical treatment in managing PMR symptoms.

Chiropractors who claim they can treat or cure PMR through spinal adjustments are not only misleading their patients but also putting them at risk of delayed or improper treatment. For patients with severe symptoms, the delay in receiving appropriate medical care can lead to prolonged suffering, worsened symptoms, and increased risk of complications such as giant cell arteritis (GCA), a serious condition often associated with PMR.

Medical treatment, including corticosteroids and physical therapy, is the most effective approach for managing PMR. While some patients may explore complementary therapies, it is crucial to recognize that chiropractic care does not address the underlying inflammatory process of PMR and could potentially do more harm than good.

Conclusion: Chiropractic Adjustments Are Not a Cure for PMR

In conclusion, while chiropractic care may be helpful for managing certain types of musculoskeletal pain, it is not an appropriate or safe treatment for Polymyalgia Rheumatica. The inflammatory process that defines PMR cannot be corrected or alleviated by spinal adjustments, and any claim to the contrary is both misleading and dangerous. Patient stories like those shared in this chapter demonstrate the very real risks of chiropractic care for PMR patients, from worsening symptoms to unnecessary delays in receiving appropriate medical treatment.

For patients with PMR, the best course of action is to seek medical treatment from specialists who understand the condition and can provide appropriate care, such as rheumatologists. Chiropractic adjustments, particularly aggressive manipulations, should be avoided due to the risk of further exacerbating muscle pain and stiffness. In the end, proper medical care—not pseudoscientific treatments—is the key to managing PMR and preventing long-term complications.

4 Cranial Therapy: Risks and Realities

In the realm of alternative medicine, cranial therapy, also known as Craniosacral Therapy (CST), is sometimes promoted as a remedy for conditions ranging from migraines to autoimmune diseases like Polymyalgia Rheumatica (PMR). Unfortunately, CST lacks any credible scientific basis, and PMR patients in particular are vulnerable to its misleading promises. CST's claims rest on dubious principles, high costs, and patient desperation, making it essential to understand why this so-called treatment not only fails to help PMR patients but can also lead to significant risks and financial strain.

What Is Cranial Therapy?

Cranial therapy purports to target and correct a non-existent "craniosacral rhythm." CST practitioners claim that this rhythm, supposedly felt through the cranial bones, influences the flow of cerebrospinal fluid (CSF) throughout the body. By applying gentle pressure on the skull, they claim they can adjust or "release" blockages, thereby improving various health issues.

However, CST's foundational beliefs are scientifically baseless. The human skull's bones fuse in adolescence, making it impossible for the cranial bones to move in any meaningful way. The idea that gentle manipulation of the skull can somehow treat PMR—a condition characterized by inflammatory pain in the muscles around the shoulders and hips—flies in the face of both anatomy and pathology. The claim that the skull needs manipulation to reduce inflammation in distant parts of the body is not only unscientific but nonsensical, especially since PMR's symptoms are caused by systemic inflammation, not mechanical blockages.

Why Do Quacks Promote CST for PMR?

For PMR patients, CST can seem appealing because of the challenges of managing the condition. PMR's symptoms—chronic pain, fatigue, and stiffness—can significantly impair daily life, and treatments like corticosteroids, while effective, come with side effects. This discomfort and the need for long-term medication make some patients receptive to "natural" alternatives that promise relief without drugs.

Quack practitioners exploit these vulnerabilities by marketing CST as a "gentle," "non-invasive" treatment option that purportedly works in harmony with the body. They claim it can alleviate inflammation and pain by releasing "blockages" in the craniosacral system, promoting general health and wellness. CST's focus on gentleness and "natural" healing makes it attractive to those who want to avoid long-term medication. Unfortunately, this approach is nothing more than pseudoscience marketed as holistic care.

Why Cranial Therapy Is Dangerous for PMR Patients

PMR is an inflammatory autoimmune condition that requires legitimate medical treatment, usually involving corticosteroids to control inflammation. For PMR patients, choosing CST over proven medical therapies can lead to several risks:

1. **Delaying or Replacing Effective Treatment**
   PMR can cause debilitating pain, reduced mobility, and, if untreated, serious complications like giant cell arteritis, which can lead to blindness. Using CST as a substitute for corticosteroids or other medications allows the disease to progress unchecked, putting patients at risk of irreversible damage.

2. **Financial Exploitation**
   CST sessions are often expensive, typically costing hundreds of dollars per session, with practitioners encouraging ongoing treatments. For PMR patients who already manage healthcare costs, these "treatments" drain financial resources without offering any actual benefit. Worse, some CST practitioners may exploit vulnerable patients by insisting that multiple sessions are necessary for results, turning CST into a high-cost commitment.

3. **Physical Harm**
   CST advocates claim their manipulations are gentle, using only five grams of pressure, but for patients with PMR, any unnecessary manipulation around the neck, shoulders, or head could exacerbate their symptoms. PMR patients often suffer severe pain and stiffness in these areas, and any additional pressure or manipulation could lead to increased discomfort or even injury. For patients with osteoporosis or other bone conditions, common among older adults with PMR, cranial manipulations can be especially risky.

The Financial Cost and Lack of Accountability in CST

One of the most striking issues with CST is its cost. CST treatments can run from $100 to $300 per session, with practitioners frequently recommending multiple sessions per week for months on end. For patients with chronic conditions, these expenses add up, creating a financial burden with no real health benefit. Moreover, CST practitioners are typically not held to the same accountability standards as licensed healthcare providers, leaving patients with limited recourse if they experience adverse effects or feel they have been misled.

Real Risks and Reported Deaths Linked to CST

While CST's claims may sound benign, its promotion has led to serious consequences. Notably, cases have emerged where reliance on CST over proper medical treatment resulted in preventable deaths. In one case, a CST practitioner convinced an epileptic patient to stop her anti-seizure medication in favor of cranial therapy, leading to fatal seizures. In another tragic instance, a practitioner performed CST on a 2-day-old infant with a high fever, resulting in the infant's death after skull manipulation.

For PMR patients, the dangers may not be as dramatic, but the risk is real: delaying effective medical care can lead to prolonged suffering, worsening symptoms, and the potential for life-altering complications. Additionally, these cases serve as reminders that CST is not only ineffective but sometimes actively harmful due to its lack of a scientific foundation.

Comparing CST to Chiropractic Adjustments

While chiropractic care and CST might seem similar because they involve physical manipulation, they differ significantly in method and theory. Chiropractic care primarily targets spinal alignment, with practitioners focusing on vertebral subluxations that they claim influence nerve function and general health. Chiropractic care has some research backing for musculoskeletal issues, though it remains controversial when applied to systemic conditions like PMR.

CST, by contrast, focuses exclusively on the skull and cerebrospinal fluid. Its practitioners claim to feel "craniosacral rhythms" and adjust them to improve health. The concept of craniosacral rhythms is scientifically unsupported, and manipulating fused skull bones is biologically implausible. PMR patients, whose primary symptoms are due to systemic inflammation, would gain no relief from spinal or cranial manipulation, as neither practice addresses the autoimmune nature of the disease.

The Scientific Consensus on Cranial Therapy

The medical and scientific communities overwhelmingly reject CST as a valid treatment. Studies have consistently failed to demonstrate the existence of "craniosacral rhythms" or measurable improvements in health outcomes from CST. Reviews, including one by the British Columbia Office of Health

Technology Assessment, have concluded that there is insufficient evidence to recommend CST as an effective therapy.

Anatomical studies also debunk CST's core premise that cranial bones move or can be manipulated to affect the entire body's health. After adolescence, cranial bones fuse, making it impossible to adjust them in the way CST claims. Furthermore, scientific attempts to measure CST's effects have shown inconsistent results, with practitioners often unable to agree on the same measurements in the same patients.

Recognizing Pseudoscience and Protecting Yourself from Quackery

For PMR patients, it's critical to differentiate evidence-based treatments from pseudoscience. Evidence-based medicine is supported by peer-reviewed research published in reputable journals, while pseudoscience relies on anecdotal claims, unverified testimonials, and marketing hype.

Reliable journals that publish research on treatments for PMR and other inflammatory diseases include:

1. *The New England Journal of Medicine*
2. *The Lancet*
3. *JAMA*
4. *Arthritis & Rheumatology*
5. *Annals of Rheumatic Diseases*

Patients are encouraged to consult with healthcare providers, check the legitimacy of treatment claims, and seek advice from reputable medical sources rather than relying on unsupported or fringe therapies like CST.

Conclusion: The Reality of CST for PMR Patients

Cranial therapy, or CST, preys on the desperation and pain of PMR patients by offering false promises under the guise of gentle, non-invasive treatment. Its core claims—that manipulating the skull can affect cerebrospinal fluid flow and treat inflammatory diseases—are unsupported by science and anatomy. For PMR patients, CST presents serious risks by delaying effective treatment, draining financial resources, and potentially worsening symptoms.

In managing PMR, it is essential to prioritize scientifically proven treatments and consult healthcare providers who rely on evidence-based approaches. PMR can be effectively managed with proper medical intervention, and the pursuit of pseudoscientific treatments like CST can undermine patients' health, finances, and hope for real relief. By understanding the science (or lack thereof) behind cranial therapy, patients can avoid falling victim to costly and dangerous quackery.

Reference:

Barrett, Stephen. "Why Cranial Therapy Is Silly." *Quackwatch*, 15 May 2004, https://quackwatch.org/related/dental-education/hcra/cranial. Accessed 24 Oct. 2024.

5 PMR Diet Myths and Facts

In alternative health circles, the idea of using diet to manage or even cure ailments has gained significant popularity. Among the more extreme claims is that a vegan or raw vegan diet can cure or dramatically improve conditions like Polymyalgia Rheumatica (PMR). While a plant-based diet offers well-documented health benefits, particularly for cardiovascular health and general wellness, the assertion that it can cure PMR is misleading and oversimplifies this complex autoimmune disorder. This chapter aims to dispel these myths while discussing how a thoughtfully planned diet can support overall health and possibly help manage some PMR symptoms, though not as a replacement for medical treatments.

Why Vegan and Raw Vegan Diets Appeal to PMR Patients

The appeal of veganism, especially raw veganism, stems from its emphasis on whole, natural foods free from animal products and processed ingredients. Proponents claim these diets reduce inflammation, lower chronic disease risks, and promote well-being. Studies indeed suggest that plant-based diets are rich in antioxidants, fiber, and essential vitamins, contributing to lower blood pressure, reduced cholesterol, and improved metabolic health.

However, the attraction of these diets for PMR patients lies in misleading claims suggesting they can alleviate or even cure PMR by reducing inflammation. This approach oversimplifies the cause of PMR, which is driven not just by inflammation but by autoimmune dysregulation, in which the immune system mistakenly attacks its own tissues. While a healthy diet can help manage some inflammatory processes, it cannot address the root cause of PMR in the immune system.

Diet Recommendations for PMR Patients

Though no diet can cure PMR, certain dietary choices may help manage inflammation and secondary health concerns associated with PMR, especially for those undergoing corticosteroid treatment, which can elevate risks for conditions like osteoporosis, weight gain, and cardiovascular disease. A balanced, anti-inflammatory diet can support overall wellness and might help alleviate some PMR symptoms, particularly by reducing systemic inflammation. Below are dietary considerations that can complement medical treatments and enhance quality of life:

1. **Anti-Inflammatory Foods**
Incorporating foods with anti-inflammatory properties can help combat pain and discomfort. Key foods include:
    - **Leafy greens** like spinach, kale, and collard greens, which are rich in antioxidants and vitamins.
    - **Berries** (such as blueberries, strawberries, and blackberries) high in fiber and antioxidants that help fight inflammation.
    - **Whole grains** like oats, quinoa, and barley, which provide fiber to help control blood sugar levels.
    - **Fatty fish** (e.g., salmon, sardines, and mackerel) for their omega-3 fatty acids, which are known to reduce inflammation. If following a vegan diet, consider omega-3 supplements or plant sources like flaxseeds, chia seeds, and walnuts.

2. **Healthy Fats**
Fats from avocados, nuts, seeds, and olive oil can help reduce inflammation and support cardiovascular health.

Extra virgin olive oil, in particular, contains oleic acid and antioxidants like polyphenols, which have been shown to help reduce markers of inflammation.

3. **Complex Carbohydrates**
Instead of refined carbohydrates (white bread, pastries, sugary cereals), focus on complex carbohydrates like sweet potatoes, brown rice, and legumes. These foods release glucose slowly into the bloodstream, reducing insulin spikes and potentially helping with energy stability throughout the day.

4. **Adequate Protein**
Protein is essential for muscle health and repair, particularly important for PMR patients who may experience muscle stiffness. Lean meats like chicken and turkey, as well as plant-based sources like beans, lentils, and tofu, are good choices.

5. **Hydration**
Staying hydrated is critical, especially as corticosteroid treatment can lead to increased thirst and fluid retention. Aim for at least 8–10 glasses of water a day, and consider incorporating herbal teas or naturally flavored water for variety.

Homocysteine Levels and Cardiovascular Risks in PMR Patients

An important consideration for PMR patients, particularly those on long-term corticosteroid therapy, is the management of homocysteine levels. Elevated homocysteine levels are linked to atherosclerosis and other cardiovascular risks, which are already a concern for those with PMR. Studies have shown that corticosteroids can increase homocysteine levels in PMR patients, adding to the need for dietary mindfulness.

B Vitamins for Homocysteine Management
A vegan diet, while beneficial in many ways, lacks certain essential nutrients, most notably vitamin B12, which is naturally found in animal products. Vitamin B12 plays a crucial role in breaking

down homocysteine. Without adequate B12, homocysteine levels can rise, increasing the risk of cardiovascular complications. PMR patients considering or following a vegan diet should ensure they supplement with B12 to mitigate this risk. Foods fortified with B12, as well as B12 supplements, are essential for vegans to prevent deficiency and its associated complications.

False Claims and Risks of a Vegan Diet for PMR

While a vegan or raw vegan diet can improve general health and provide anti-inflammatory benefits, no diet can cure or reverse PMR. PMR's symptoms result from an autoimmune process that attacks the body's own tissues. Diet alone cannot regulate or reverse this immune response. The only proven treatments for PMR include corticosteroids and other immune-modulating medications.

Despite these facts, misinformation about diet-based "cures" for PMR abounds, often claiming that raw or vegan diets can detoxify the body and "reset" the immune system. While these diets may appeal to those seeking non-drug solutions, they cannot replace the need for corticosteroids in managing PMR's progression and symptoms. Worse, if patients forgo medical treatments in favor of unproven diets, they risk exacerbating their symptoms or experiencing serious complications.

Practical Diet Guidelines for PMR Patients

A balanced approach is ideal for PMR patients seeking dietary support. Here are practical guidelines that emphasize both nutritional balance and managing inflammation:

1. **The Mediterranean Diet**
   Known for its heart-healthy benefits, the Mediterranean diet emphasizes fresh fruits, vegetables, whole grains, and healthy fats, along with moderate portions of lean proteins like fish and poultry. This diet is naturally anti-inflammatory, rich in antioxidants, and supports heart health, making it particularly suitable for PMR patients who need to manage inflammation and reduce cardiovascular risk.

2. **A Modified Plant-Based Diet**
   While a strict vegan diet may not be necessary or suitable for all PMR patients, a modified plant-based approach that includes lean animal proteins can provide a balance of nutrients. This diet emphasizes plant foods while incorporating fish, eggs, and occasionally lean meats. This flexibility ensures patients get enough B12, iron, and protein, reducing the need for heavy supplementation.

3. **Anti-Inflammatory Diet Principles**
   Similar to the Mediterranean diet, an anti-inflammatory diet focuses on vegetables, fruits, whole grains, lean proteins, and healthy fats. Avoiding added sugars, processed foods, and refined carbohydrates is crucial, as these foods can trigger inflammatory processes. Including foods rich in omega-3s, like chia seeds or walnuts, can help manage inflammation without compromising on taste or nutrition.

4. **Portion Control and Regular Meals**
   Regular, well-balanced meals help maintain stable blood sugar levels and reduce fatigue. Patients might find it helpful to have smaller, balanced meals every 3–4 hours rather than larger, less frequent meals to maintain energy levels throughout the day.

5. **Bone Health and Calcium-Rich Foods**
   Since corticosteroids can weaken bones, PMR patients should aim to consume adequate calcium and vitamin D. Dairy products, leafy greens, and fortified plant-based milks can all contribute to bone health. Calcium and vitamin D supplements may be necessary for those who cannot meet their daily needs through diet alone, particularly in vegan diets.

Conclusion: Adopting a Realistic and Supportive Diet

For PMR patients, dietary choices play a supportive role in managing symptoms and promoting overall health, but they are not a replacement for medical treatments. While diets like veganism or raw veganism may appeal to those looking for alternative treatments, they cannot address the autoimmune mechanisms underlying PMR. A balanced approach—focused on anti-inflammatory, nutrient-rich foods—can, however, complement conventional treatments and provide additional health benefits.

PMR patients are encouraged to adopt a realistic view of what diet can and cannot do. By following an anti-inflammatory diet, rich in plant-based foods and healthy fats, they can improve their quality of life, reduce inflammation, and manage secondary symptoms like cardiovascular risk. Supplementation with vitamin B12 is essential for those who choose a plant-based diet, as are calcium and vitamin D if corticosteroids are part of the treatment plan.

Ultimately, a tailored diet, informed by medical advice, can be a valuable part of an overall PMR management plan, helping patients feel more in control of their health without falling for the false promise of a "cure" through diet alone.

Reference:

V. M. Martinez-Taboada, M. J. Bartolome, M. D. Fernandez-Gonzalez, R. Blanco, V. Rodriguez-Valverde, M. Lopez-Hoyos, Homocysteine levels in polymyalgia rheumatica and giant cell arteritis: influence of corticosteroid therapy, *Rheumatology*, Volume 42, Issue 9, September 2003, Pages 1055–1061, https://doi.org/10.1093/rheumatology/keg293

6 Other Pseudoscientific Diets

The alkaline diet is based on the idea that certain foods can affect the acidity or alkalinity (pH) of the body's fluids, particularly the blood, and that consuming more alkaline foods can help prevent or even reverse diseases like Polymyalgia Rheumatica (PMR). However, this notion is grounded in pseudoscience and is not supported by any credible evidence in the medical literature. While a diet rich in fruits and vegetables can improve overall health, there is no scientifically sound evidence to suggest that it can cure or alleviate the symptoms of PMR, an autoimmune condition.

In addition to the alkaline diet, there are several other pseudoscientific diets that make false claims about curing or managing complex autoimmune conditions like PMR. The raw food diet, for example, is often promoted as a way to "detox" the body and heal chronic conditions, yet there is no scientific evidence that eating only raw foods can cure autoimmune conditions. Another popular pseudoscientific diet is the carnivore diet, which advocates eating only meat and animal products. Proponents of this diet claim it can reduce inflammation and even cure autoimmune diseases, but again, no credible medical literature supports these claims. Other extreme diets, such as juice cleanses or fasting regimens, are marketed as ways to "reset" the body's immune system, but they lack scientific validity and can lead to dangerous nutrient deficiencies. These diets, like the alkaline diet, mislead patients into believing that radical dietary changes can resolve serious medical conditions, often delaying or replacing necessary medical treatment.

The problem with such diets is that they promise cures based on false premises and mislead vulnerable patients who are desperate for solutions. In this chapter, we will explore the pseudoscientific foundation of the alkaline diet, discuss how credibility is determined in medical research, and explain how patients can ensure that the diets they choose are backed by sound science.

The Alkaline Diet: Misunderstanding Human Physiology

The premise of the alkaline diet is that certain foods can change the pH of the body and make it less acidic. Advocates of the diet claim that a more alkaline environment in the body can prevent or even cure various diseases, including cancer, arthritis, and autoimmune conditions like PMR. However, this claim ignores basic human physiology.

The human body tightly regulates its pH levels, especially in the blood. The normal pH of blood ranges from 7.35 to 7.45, and the body has several mechanisms, including kidney function and respiratory control, to keep it within this range. This regulation is crucial for survival, and no amount of dietary change can significantly alter blood pH in a healthy person. If the body's pH were to shift outside this narrow range, it would indicate a serious medical condition, such as acidosis or alkalosis, which requires immediate medical intervention—not a dietary change.

While it's true that certain foods can temporarily change the pH of urine, this does not reflect a change in the body's overall pH. In fact, this urinary change is part of the body's natural process to maintain the balance of blood pH. The idea that diet alone can "balance" the body's pH and cure autoimmune conditions like PMR is not only incorrect but potentially harmful.

Lack of Credible Support: What It Really Means

The alkaline diet, like many other pseudoscientific health fads, lacks credible support in the medical literature. But what exactly does "credible" mean in this context? To understand this, we need to look at how scientific credibility is measured.

In the medical and scientific community, the credibility of research is determined by several factors:

1. **Peer Review Process**: Credible studies are published in peer-reviewed journals. In this process, research is evaluated by independent experts in the same field who assess the study's methodology, data, and conclusions to ensure they are sound and unbiased. This vetting process is designed to catch errors, prevent bias, and ensure that only valid research is published. If a claim, such as the idea that the alkaline diet can cure PMR, is not supported by peer-reviewed research, it should be viewed with skepticism.

2. **Reproducibility of Results**: For a study to be considered credible, its results must be reproducible. This means that other researchers should be able to conduct the same experiment and achieve the same results. If a claim about a diet's effectiveness is based on a single study or anecdotal evidence, and it cannot be replicated, it is not considered credible.

3. **Sample Size and Control Groups**: Credible research involves large enough sample sizes to ensure the findings are not due to chance. It also includes control groups to compare results and rule out other factors. Many of the studies supporting diets like the alkaline diet are either based on very small sample sizes or lack control groups, which undermines their validity.

4. **Absence of Bias**: Scientific credibility also depends on the absence of financial or personal bias. Studies funded by parties with vested interests, such as companies selling supplements or diet plans, may be biased toward producing favorable results. Credible research is transparent about its funding and potential conflicts of

interest.

5. **Plausibility Based on Established Science**: For a new claim to be credible, it must make sense in the context of existing scientific knowledge. The alkaline diet's premise—that foods can significantly alter blood pH and affect disease outcomes—is implausible based on what we know about human physiology and biochemistry.

How to Identify Peer-Reviewed Research

For patients who are not familiar with scientific research, identifying credible sources can be challenging. Here are a few ways to ensure that the information you're considering has scientific backing:

1. **Look for Peer-Reviewed Journals**: Peer-reviewed journals are the gold standard for reliable scientific information. Journals like *The New England Journal of Medicine*, *The Lancet*, and *The Journal of Nutrition* only publish studies that have been reviewed by experts in the field. To verify that a study has been peer-reviewed, you can search for it on databases like PubMed, which only indexes research from reputable, peer-reviewed sources.

2. **Consult Meta-Analyses and Systematic Reviews**: These types of research synthesize the findings of multiple studies, providing a more comprehensive overview of a topic. If a diet like the alkaline diet were truly effective, there would be numerous high-quality studies supporting it, and these would be summarized in meta-analyses or systematic reviews.

3. **Watch Out for Red Flags**: Be skeptical of health claims that are based on anecdotal evidence, personal testimonials, or claims of a "miracle cure." Diets that promise to cure serious conditions like PMR are almost always too good to be true.

4. **Trusted Medical Sources**: Government health agencies such as the National Institutes of Health (NIH), the

Centers for Disease Control and Prevention (CDC), and the World Health Organization (WHO) provide reliable, science-backed information on diets and health. Additionally, reputable medical organizations like the Mayo Clinic and Cleveland Clinic offer trustworthy dietary advice.

A List of Peer-Reviewed Journals on Diet and Nutrition

Here are a few examples of reputable, peer-reviewed journals that regularly publish research on nutrition and diet:

- *The American Journal of Clinical Nutrition*
- *The Journal of Nutrition*
- *Nutrition Reviews*
- *The British Journal of Nutrition*
- *The Journal of the Academy of Nutrition and Dietetics*
- *Public Health Nutrition*
- *Nutrition and Metabolism*

These journals are excellent sources for reliable information about the health effects of various diets. If a diet is truly beneficial for health, you will find studies supporting it in journals like these, rather than on blogs or in books written by non-experts.

Why Are Pseudoscientific Diets Like the Alkaline Diet So Popular?

Despite the lack of credible evidence, diets like the alkaline diet continue to be popular, especially among patients with chronic conditions. There are several reasons for this:

1. **Desperation for Relief**: Patients with chronic illnesses, like PMR, often experience long-term symptoms that conventional treatments cannot fully resolve. The promise of a dietary cure, even if it's not scientifically supported, can seem like a beacon of hope.

2. **Appeal of Natural Remedies**: Many pseudoscientific diets market themselves as "natural" solutions, which appeals to individuals who are wary of pharmaceuticals or surgery. The idea that health can be restored through natural foods is enticing, even though not all "natural" approaches are effective or safe.

3. **Mistrust of Conventional Medicine**: Some patients turn to alternative diets because they feel that conventional medicine has failed them or because they mistrust the pharmaceutical industry. In such cases, pseudoscientific diets can seem like a safer, more holistic alternative.

4. **Persuasive Marketing**: The marketing behind pseudoscientific diets is often very persuasive, using emotional appeals and personal testimonials to draw people in. Unfortunately, these claims are rarely backed by sound science.

5. **Confirmation Bias**: Once a person adopts a pseudoscientific diet and feels better—perhaps due to unrelated lifestyle changes or a placebo effect—they may attribute their improvement to the diet, reinforcing their belief in its effectiveness even without scientific evidence.

Ensuring Credibility When Choosing a Diet

For patients, especially those with chronic conditions like PMR, it's critical to ensure that the diet they choose is supported by credible, peer-reviewed research. While adopting a plant-based diet can have many health benefits, it's essential to be aware of the pseudoscientific claims surrounding diets like the alkaline diet. By focusing on diets that are based on sound science and paying attention to credible research, patients can make informed decisions that promote their overall well-being without falling prey to false claims.

7 Diluting Reality

Homeopathy is a widely criticized and scientifically disproven system of alternative medicine that is based on two main principles: like cures like and extreme dilution. Although it continues to be a popular alternative therapy, particularly among those suffering from chronic conditions, it has no place in treating autoimmune and inflammatory disorders like Polymyalgia Rheumatica (PMR).

PMR is an inflammatory condition that primarily affects the muscles, causing stiffness, pain, and significant discomfort, particularly in the shoulders and hips. This is a systemic issue that stems from inflammation, and not one that can be addressed by remedies relying on diluting substances to the point of being essentially non-existent, as is the case with homeopathy. Yet, despite the lack of scientific evidence, some homeopaths make bold claims about their ability to relieve the symptoms of PMR.

In this chapter, we will delve into the foundations of homeopathy, discuss why homeopathic treatments are ineffective for conditions like PMR, and highlight patient stories that show the dangers of choosing homeopathy over scientifically proven treatments.

The Appeal of Homeopathy for PMR Patients

Homeopathy has remained popular for over two centuries, even as modern medicine has advanced significantly. Part of its enduring appeal lies in its perceived safety—homeopathic remedies are often marketed as "natural," "gentle," and "free from side effects." Many people with chronic or poorly understood conditions, like PMR, may feel disillusioned with conventional medical treatments, particularly when those treatments involve long-term steroid use, potential side effects, or lifestyle changes that can be difficult to manage. Homeopathy, with its promise of a gentle, holistic cure, can be an alluring option.

Additionally, homeopathic practitioners tend to spend a great deal of time with their patients, offering empathy, attention, and a personalized approach to care. This contrasts with the often rushed and clinical environment of conventional medicine, particularly for conditions like PMR, where patients may see multiple specialists and endure lengthy waiting periods between appointments. The combination of personal attention, the promise of a simple cure, and frustration with conventional treatments can lead patients toward homeopathy, even when it is ineffective or potentially harmful.

The Dangers of Homeopathy for PMR

While the appeal of homeopathy is understandable, the dangers are significant. PMR is an inflammatory condition, and homeopathy cannot address the systemic inflammation driving the symptoms. Homeopathy is based on principles that defy basic science, and relying on it as a treatment for PMR can have serious consequences.

One of the biggest dangers of homeopathy is the delay it causes in receiving appropriate treatment. PMR is typically managed with corticosteroids, which reduce inflammation and provide significant relief from symptoms. Left untreated, PMR can worsen, leading to increased pain, stiffness, and potentially complicating the patient's condition with other inflammatory diseases such as giant cell arteritis (GCA), which can cause irreversible vision loss. Homeopathy, with its reliance on highly diluted substances with no active ingredients, cannot reduce the inflammation driving PMR symptoms, and delaying corticosteroid treatment in favor of homeopathic remedies can lead to significant harm.

Consider the case of James, a 65-year-old man diagnosed with PMR after experiencing months of stiffness and pain. Fearful of the potential side effects of steroids, James turned to a homeopath who promised that a series of diluted remedies could cure his condition. After spending a year on these treatments, James' symptoms had not improved, and he began to experience severe vision problems—a complication from undiagnosed GCA. By the time he sought conventional medical treatment, it was too late to reverse the vision loss, and he now lives with permanent blindness in one eye. His delay in seeking proper treatment caused irreversible damage.

James' story is not unique. Many PMR patients turn to homeopathy in the hope of avoiding medications with side effects or because they believe in the body's ability to heal itself. However, in the case of PMR, where inflammation must be actively managed to prevent complications, there is no alternative to medical intervention, whether through steroids or other immunosuppressive medications. The inflammatory nature of PMR cannot be corrected through diluted remedies that lack any active ingredient.

Why Homeopathy Cannot Address Inflammatory Conditions Like PMR

One of the central claims of homeopathy is that "like cures like"—that is, a substance that causes symptoms in a healthy person can cure those same symptoms in a sick person when diluted to extreme levels. For example, homeopaths might suggest that a diluted solution of a substance that causes joint pain could cure PMR-related joint pain. However, this principle does not hold up to scientific scrutiny. Homeopathic remedies are so diluted that they contain no molecules of the original substance, and numerous studies have shown that they are no more effective than placebos.

Even if homeopathy could somehow trigger a healing response for minor ailments (which it does not), it still would not be capable of addressing the systemic inflammation involved in PMR. The core issue in PMR is widespread inflammation in the muscles and joints, driven by the immune system. No amount of diluted substances can reduce this inflammation or relieve the pain and stiffness associated with it.

Homeopathic practitioners may claim that their remedies can relieve PMR symptoms like muscle stiffness or fatigue, but these claims are unsupported by any credible evidence. While patients may experience temporary relief through the placebo effect, this is not a true resolution of the underlying condition, and the symptoms will inevitably return or worsen without proper treatment. For PMR patients, delaying effective treatment can lead to unnecessary pain and complications, and the reliance on homeopathy is, therefore, a dangerous gamble.

Guy Chapman's Critique of Homeopathy

In his submission to a U.K. Parliamentary Committee, Guy Chapman presents a comprehensive critique of the false claims made by homeopathy proponents. His arguments are particularly relevant to patients with conditions like PMR, as they highlight the dangers of relying on pseudoscientific treatments that lack credible evidence. Chapman's key points further dismantle the myth that homeopathy can cure or alleviate serious conditions, underscoring the importance of evidence-based medicine.

Chapman draws attention to several major issues within the homeopathy community, starting with the frequent misrepresentation of sources. One of the central examples he cites is the "Health Technology Assessment" (HTA), which was presented by homeopaths as a legitimate, government-backed study. However, Chapman reveals that this so-called HTA was not a true scientific review, but rather a biased and reworked version of a previously failed submission to the Swiss Government's complementary medicine evaluation program. Not only was this document falsely labeled as an HTA, but it was also riddled with conflicts of interest that undermine its credibility.

For PMR patients, this example is particularly relevant. It demonstrates how proponents of homeopathy and similar alternative therapies may distort or manipulate evidence to support their claims. The reality, as Chapman and the original Swiss review revealed, is that homeopathy has no demonstrated effect beyond placebo for any medical condition. This fact is vital for PMR patients to understand, as homeopathy's lack of effectiveness could delay the appropriate diagnosis and treatment of serious symptoms.

Chapman also delves into the broader body of scientific evidence on homeopathy. He references a meta-analysis commissioned by the Swiss program, which was later published in *The Lancet*, that found no compelling evidence that homeopathy worked better than placebo. Furthermore, Chapman explains that the few positive results that have emerged from homeopathic studies tend to be associated with weaker research methodologies. In other words, the more rigorously a study is designed, the less likely it is to show any benefit from homeopathic treatments. This is crucial for PMR patients, as it underscores that the apparent "effectiveness" of homeopathy in some cases is not due to the treatment itself, but rather to flawed research or placebo effects.

Moreover, Chapman emphasizes that the use of homeopathy in cases where effective medical treatments exist can be unethical and dangerous. He gives the example of using homeopathy to treat upper respiratory infections (URTIs) or ear infections (acute otitis media, or AOM). While homeopaths may claim that their remedies can replace antibiotics, Chapman explains that this is misleading, as most URTIs and AOM cases resolve on their own. The danger lies in patients mistaking the natural course of an illness for the effectiveness of a homeopathic remedy. This risk is particularly relevant to PMR patients, whose condition can lead to persistent inflammation and pain that require careful medical management. By relying on homeopathy instead of seeking proper treatment, patients could face worsening symptoms or long-term damage.

Patient Stories: False Hope and Real Harm

In addition to James' case, many other PMR patients have turned to homeopathy in the hope of finding relief, only to be disappointed by the lack of results. In some cases, patients have spent thousands of dollars on homeopathic treatments over the course of months or even years, only to find themselves in worse condition than when they started.

Take the story of Sarah, a 58-year-old woman diagnosed with PMR. She had been managing her symptoms with corticosteroids for several months but was concerned about the long-term side effects of these medications. After reading about homeopathy online, she decided to give it a try, despite her doctor's recommendation to continue her current treatment. Over the course of six months, Sarah's homeopath prescribed a variety of remedies, including diluted solutions of various plants and minerals. At first, Sarah thought she felt better, but this was likely the placebo effect at work. Eventually, her symptoms—muscle stiffness, fatigue, and joint pain—became so severe that she could barely move. When she finally returned to her doctor, it became clear that her condition had worsened significantly, and she had to restart steroid treatment immediately.

Sarah's story illustrates the false hope that homeopathy offers. Patients are led to believe that they are receiving treatment when, in reality, they are receiving nothing more than sugar pills and water. The time and money spent on homeopathy are wasted, and the patient's health continues to deteriorate while they chase an impossible cure.

Conclusion: Diluting Reality

In conclusion, homeopathy is based on principles that have no scientific foundation. According to the National Center for Complementary and Integrative Health (NCCIH), which is part of the U.S. National Institutes of Health, "There is little evidence to support homeopathy as an effective treatment for any specific condition" and "several key concepts of homeopathy are inconsistent with fundamental concepts of chemistry and physics."

For conditions like PMR, which involve systemic inflammation, homeopathic remedies are not just ineffective—

they are dangerously misleading. The false hope they offer can delay effective treatment, leading to unnecessary suffering and potential complications. While homeopathy may seem like a gentle, natural alternative to conventional medication, it is nothing more than a placebo, and it has no place in the treatment of PMR.

References:

Chapman, Guy. "Written Evidence Submitted by Guy Chapman (AMR0058)." *Parliament UK*, 17 Dec. 2012, https://committees.parliament.uk/writtenevidence/48855/html/.

National Center for Complementary and Integrative Health. "Homeopathy." *NCCIH*, U.S. Department of Health and Human Services, Aug. 2016, www.nccih.nih.gov/health/homeopathy.

8 Energy Healing: Promises Without Proof

Energy healing, which encompasses practices like Reiki, Therapeutic Touch, and Qi Gong, is often marketed as a gentle, non-invasive way to alleviate a variety of ailments. Practitioners claim to manipulate or balance a person's "life energy" to promote healing and relieve symptoms. These therapies often involve no physical contact, instead relying on the belief that the practitioner can direct healing energy into or around the patient's body. For patients with autoimmune conditions like Polymyalgia Rheumatica (PMR), this form of treatment is sometimes suggested as a way to alleviate symptoms such as muscle pain, stiffness, or fatigue. However, while energy healing may seem appealing due to its non-invasive nature, it is a practice with no scientific backing, posing particular dangers for individuals with serious health conditions like PMR.

In this chapter, we will explore the pseudoscientific foundations of energy healing practices like Reiki, the difference between patient testimonials and actual clinical outcomes, and the dangers posed by these therapies for those suffering from autoimmune conditions. We will also delve into how the placebo effect plays a crucial role in any perceived benefits and why relying on such treatments can be both misleading and risky for PMR patients.

The Pseudoscientific Foundation of Energy Healing

Energy healing is based on the concept of "life energy" or "vital energy" that flows through and around the human body. Different cultures have had their own interpretations of this energy, such as qi in Chinese medicine, prana in Hinduism, and ki in the Japanese practice of Reiki. The fundamental belief is that when this energy becomes blocked or imbalanced, it can cause physical or emotional illness. Energy healers claim they can manipulate this energy, either by laying their hands on or near the patient's body, to restore balance and, in turn, alleviate symptoms.

Reiki, one of the most well-known forms of energy healing, was developed in Japan by Mikao Usui in the early 20th century. Usui claimed that Reiki practitioners could channel healing energy from a universal source through their hands into the patient, promoting healing and well-being. Today, Reiki has become a popular form of alternative therapy, often advertised as a way to relieve stress, improve overall health, and in some cases, treat serious conditions like PMR.

However, the idea of manipulating an invisible energy field remains unsupported by modern science. The human body does not contain any measurable "energy fields" that could be altered to improve health. Moreover, there is no scientific evidence to suggest that Reiki or any other form of energy healing has any effect beyond the placebo response. The principles upon which energy healing is based are incompatible with well-established scientific knowledge about biology and physics, which makes it a pseudoscientific practice.

Testimonials Versus Actual Outcomes

One of the reasons energy healing has remained popular is the abundance of glowing testimonials from patients who claim to have benefited from it. These individuals often report feeling more relaxed, experiencing reduced pain, or having an improved sense of well-being after receiving energy healing treatments. Such accounts can be compelling, especially for patients who are struggling to find relief through conventional medical treatments.

However, patient testimonials, no matter how sincere, are not the same as scientifically verified outcomes. Anecdotal evidence is subjective and prone to bias. People may attribute improvement in their condition to energy healing, when in fact other factors may be at play, such as natural recovery over time, the placebo effect, or even a desire to believe in the efficacy of the treatment due to the financial or emotional investment they have made.

In scientific research, the effectiveness of a treatment is determined through rigorous testing, such as randomized controlled trials (RCTs), where treatments are compared to a placebo in a controlled environment. To date, no high-quality clinical trials have demonstrated that energy healing practices like Reiki provide any therapeutic benefits beyond placebo. While some studies suggest that patients report feeling better after a Reiki session, these results can be explained by the placebo effect, rather than by any real manipulation of life energy.

Why Energy Healing is Dangerous for Patients with PMR

For individuals with autoimmune conditions like PMR, relying on energy healing can be particularly dangerous. PMR is characterized by widespread muscle pain and stiffness, primarily affecting the shoulders and hips. Without proper treatment, the condition can lead to severe pain, reduced mobility, and in some cases, complications such as giant cell arteritis (GCA), which can cause vision loss. PMR often requires corticosteroids or other anti-inflammatory medications to control inflammation and prevent further damage. Energy healing cannot reduce this inflammation or address the immune system's overactivity.

One of the risks of energy healing is that it may give patients a false sense of security. If someone with PMR believes that their symptoms are improving due to Reiki sessions, they may delay seeking appropriate medical care. For example, they might forgo recommended medications or physical therapy that could genuinely improve their condition. As PMR symptoms worsen, untreated, patients could face more pain and long-term mobility issues.

Another danger lies in the lack of regulation within the energy healing field. Practitioners of Reiki or other forms of energy healing are not required to undergo medical training or certification in most regions, meaning that anyone can claim to be an energy healer. Patients with PMR or other serious health conditions are vulnerable to being exploited by practitioners who make false claims about their abilities to heal or alleviate symptoms. This lack of regulation leaves patients without any recourse should they be harmed, financially or otherwise, by these treatments.

The Placebo Effect in Energy Healing

One of the key factors that keeps energy healing practices like Reiki alive despite the lack of scientific evidence is the placebo effect. The placebo effect occurs when a patient experiences an improvement in their symptoms simply because they believe they are receiving treatment, even if the treatment itself has no therapeutic value. The human brain is powerful, and belief in a treatment, even a pseudoscientific one, can lead to real changes in how a patient feels.

In the context of energy healing, the placebo effect can be particularly strong. The calm, relaxing environment of a Reiki session, combined with the soothing presence of the practitioner, can induce feelings of relaxation and stress relief, which can make patients feel temporarily better. This improvement is not due to any manipulation of life energy but rather to the psychological benefits of feeling cared for and engaged in a healing process.

For patients with PMR, the placebo effect may lead to temporary relief of symptoms such as anxiety or tension, but it will not address the underlying inflammation causing their pain and stiffness. Relying on placebo-driven relief may delay proper medical intervention, which is crucial for managing a progressive condition like PMR.

While the placebo effect may offer some short-term psychological benefits, it is not a replacement for evidence-based medical care. Patients with serious health conditions should be wary of treatments that rely solely on the placebo effect without offering any real therapeutic benefits.

Energy Healing and the "Healing" Industry

The rise of energy healing can be seen as part of a broader trend in the alternative health industry, where treatments are marketed as holistic and natural alternatives to conventional medicine. This industry often appeals to patients who feel disillusioned by the medical establishment or who are seeking treatments for conditions that are difficult to manage, such as chronic pain or autoimmune disorders.

For PMR patients, who often experience debilitating pain and stiffness, the allure of a simple, non-invasive treatment like energy healing can be particularly strong. Practitioners of Reiki and other forms of energy healing may prey on these vulnerabilities by promising to relieve symptoms without the need for medications or other interventions. However, these promises are empty, and they are not supported by any credible scientific evidence.

Patients with PMR should approach any treatment that claims to offer a cure or significant relief with skepticism, especially if the treatment is not backed by clinical research. While energy healing may seem harmless on the surface, the financial and emotional costs of investing in pseudoscientific therapies can be high, particularly when they distract patients from seeking effective medical treatments.

Conclusion

Energy healing practices like Reiki, which claim to manipulate a person's life energy to relieve symptoms, are based on pseudoscientific principles that lack any real grounding in biology or medicine. For patients with serious autoimmune conditions like PMR, relying on such treatments can be dangerous, as it may delay appropriate medical care and leave symptoms untreated. The perceived benefits of energy healing are largely driven by the placebo effect, which can provide short-term psychological relief but will not address the underlying inflammation causing PMR symptoms.

It is crucial for PMR patients to be informed about the lack of evidence supporting energy healing and to make treatment decisions based on scientific research and the advice of medical professionals. While energy healing may seem like a gentle, non-invasive option, it is ultimately a distraction from the real, evidence-based treatments that PMR patients need to manage their condition effectively.

9 Flushing Out False Hopes

In recent years, detox and cleansing therapies have gained immense popularity in alternative medicine circles. Promoters of these therapies claim that a wide variety of ailments, from digestive disorders to autoimmune conditions like Polymyalgia Rheumatica (PMR), can be alleviated or even cured by ridding the body of so-called "toxins." Whether it's liver cleanses, colon cleanses, juice fasts, or special detox diets, these approaches are touted as magical remedies for everything under the sun. Unfortunately, while these detox methods might sound appealing to individuals suffering from chronic conditions like PMR, they are based on pseudoscientific principles and offer false hope. In this chapter, we will explore the myths surrounding detox and cleansing therapies, explain why these treatments are dangerous for individuals with autoimmune conditions like PMR, and discuss how the placebo effect plays a significant role in perceived benefits.

The Myth of Detoxification

Detox and cleansing therapies are built on the premise that the body is full of harmful toxins that accumulate over time and cause disease. According to proponents of these methods, toxins come from various sources: pollution, pesticides, processed foods, alcohol, heavy metals, medications, and even stress. By undergoing a cleanse, patients are promised that these toxins will be flushed from their bodies, restoring balance and health. However, the fundamental problem with this premise is that there is no scientific evidence to support the idea that our bodies are "toxic" in this way, nor is there any proof that detox diets or cleanses can remove harmful substances from the body.

The human body is remarkably efficient at detoxifying itself. The liver, kidneys, lungs, skin, and gastrointestinal tract work together to process and eliminate waste products and toxins every day. The liver metabolizes harmful substances and breaks them down into less toxic forms, while the kidneys filter the blood and excrete waste through urine. The lungs expel carbon dioxide, and the skin eliminates waste through sweat. In short, the body already has a highly effective built-in detoxification system. Claims that detox diets or cleanses can do a better job of purifying the body are both misleading and scientifically unfounded.

Most detox diets and cleanses involve extreme measures such as fasting, drinking only juice for extended periods, or taking herbal supplements that are supposed to stimulate the liver or colon. While these practices might make people feel as though they are doing something proactive for their health, they often have little to no real impact on the body's natural detoxification processes. Moreover, detox diets can have serious negative side effects, especially for people with pre-existing conditions like PMR.

Why Detox Therapies Are Dangerous for PMR Patients

Polymyalgia Rheumatica is an autoimmune condition that causes widespread muscle pain, stiffness, and inflammation, primarily affecting the shoulders, neck, and hips. PMR is typically managed through the use of corticosteroids to reduce inflammation, along with other anti-inflammatory medications. Detox and cleansing therapies, however, do nothing to address the underlying autoimmune dysfunction that causes PMR symptoms. The idea that flushing the colon or drinking detox juices can reduce inflammation in the muscles or improve immune function is patently absurd.

What makes these therapies especially dangerous for PMR patients is the potential for dehydration, electrolyte imbalances, and nutrient deficiencies, which can exacerbate symptoms. For example, many detox diets recommend extreme calorie restriction, juice fasting, or consuming only certain "cleansing" foods for days or even weeks at a time. These practices can deprive the body of essential nutrients, weaken the immune system, and lead to physical exhaustion. PMR patients, who may already experience fatigue, muscle weakness, and pain, are at greater risk of these side effects. Severe dehydration or electrolyte imbalances can also worsen fatigue, confusion, and muscle cramping—symptoms that are already common in PMR patients.

Additionally, some detox regimens include herbal supplements that claim to "flush out" the liver or colon. Many of these supplements are unregulated, and their safety and efficacy have not been proven. Some contain powerful laxatives or diuretics, which can lead to diarrhea, cramping, and dehydration. PMR patients, who often require careful management of their symptoms and medication regimens, could face severe complications from such drastic methods.

Colon Cleansing: A Dangerous Trend

One of the most dangerous trends in the detox world is colon cleansing. Proponents claim that toxins build up in the colon over time and need to be flushed out to improve overall health. This idea, sometimes referred to as "autointoxication," is based on the long-debunked theory that waste material in the colon can be reabsorbed into the bloodstream, causing a wide range of health problems. Colon cleansing procedures—often involving enemas, colonic irrigation, or herbal laxatives—are promoted as a way to remove these toxins and restore health.

For PMR patients, colon cleansing is particularly hazardous. First, there is no credible scientific evidence that the colon requires cleansing. The body is fully capable of expelling waste naturally through normal bowel movements, and there is no need to flush the colon unless directed by a healthcare provider for medical reasons (such as before a colonoscopy). Secondly, the risks associated with colon cleansing include dehydration, electrolyte imbalances, infections, perforation of the colon, and bowel damage. These risks can be life-threatening, particularly for individuals with pre-existing conditions like PMR.

Juice Fasting: Nutrient Deficiency and Fatigue

Juice fasting is another common detox method promoted as a way to "cleanse" the body of toxins. Typically, juice fasts involve consuming only fruit and vegetable juices for several days or weeks. Advocates claim that this gives the digestive system a break, allowing the body to focus on healing itself. They also claim that juice fasts flood the body with vitamins and antioxidants, promoting better health.

While it's true that fruits and vegetables are packed with essential nutrients, juice fasting can deprive the body of important macronutrients like protein and fat, which are necessary for energy production and muscle maintenance. For PMR patients, who may already suffer from fatigue and muscle weakness, going on a juice fast could lead to even greater weakness, dizziness, and cognitive impairment. Prolonged juice fasting can also result in dangerous drops in blood sugar, which can exacerbate fatigue, muscle pain, and other PMR symptoms.

Additionally, juice fasts can be high in sugar, particularly if they rely heavily on fruit juices. High sugar intake can cause spikes and crashes in blood sugar levels, leading to mood swings, irritability, and fatigue—symptoms that can overlap with or worsen the pain and stiffness of PMR.

Why People Believe in Detox and Cleansing Therapies

Despite the lack of scientific evidence supporting detox and cleansing therapies, many people continue to believe in their efficacy. One reason is the seductive simplicity of the detox narrative: the idea that poor health is caused by toxins and that these toxins can be easily removed through a cleanse appeals to people who are desperate for quick and easy solutions. For patients with chronic conditions like PMR, who often face limited treatment options and frustratingly slow progress, the promise of detox as a cure-all is especially enticing.

Testimonials play a huge role in perpetuating the belief in detox therapies. Individuals who undergo a cleanse often report feeling better afterward, attributing their improved sense of well-being to the removal of toxins. However, in most cases, these improvements can be explained by the placebo effect, changes in diet (such as temporarily cutting out processed foods), or simply the body's natural ability to recover after short-term fasting or rest. The placebo effect is particularly strong in cases where patients have faith in the detox process and believe that it will help them.

Another reason why detox therapies are so popular is the marketing tactics used by the wellness industry. Companies that sell detox supplements, juices, and programs often employ fear-based messaging, warning people about the dangers of toxins and emphasizing the need for constant detoxification. This fear, combined with the allure of quick results, drives people to purchase detox products, despite the lack of evidence supporting their effectiveness.

The Placebo Effect and Perceived Benefits

One of the most compelling reasons why people continue to turn to detox and cleansing therapies is the placebo effect. The placebo effect occurs when a person experiences a perceived improvement in symptoms simply because they believe a treatment is working, even if the treatment itself has no therapeutic value. In the case of detox therapies, the act of doing something proactive for one's health—whether it's drinking juice, taking supplements, or undergoing a cleanse—can make people feel better psychologically, even if there is no real physical benefit.

The placebo effect is powerful, and it can lead to genuine improvements in mood, energy levels, and overall well-being. However, for PMR patients, relying on the placebo effect to manage serious autoimmune symptoms is risky. While a patient might feel temporarily better after a detox or cleanse, the underlying inflammation and muscle stiffness remain untreated, and important medical interventions might be delayed.

Conclusion: Detoxing from Detox Myths

Detox and cleansing therapies are built on a pseudoscientific foundation that misleads patients into believing that toxins are responsible for their health problems. For individuals with autoimmune conditions like PMR, these therapies offer false hope and can even be dangerous. PMR is an inflammatory condition that cannot be "flushed away" through fasting, colon cleansing, or detox supplements. Proper medical treatment, including the use of corticosteroids and anti-inflammatory medications, is essential for managing PMR symptoms and preventing complications.

10 Misleading Nature's Potential

Herbal remedies have been a cornerstone of traditional medicine for centuries, with plants and herbs being used to treat various ailments long before modern pharmaceuticals existed. Some of these herbs have well-documented benefits, such as ginger for nausea or echinacea for immune support. However, when it comes to autoimmune conditions like Polymyalgia Rheumatica (PMR), the use of herbal remedies strays into dangerous territory. While many people assume that because something is "natural," it must be safe and effective, this chapter explores the reality that not all herbs are beneficial, especially for complex medical conditions like PMR. More importantly, the claims that herbal remedies can treat or cure PMR are unsubstantiated and, in some cases, harmful.

The Appeal of Herbal Remedies for Chronic Conditions

Herbal medicine is often appealing to patients because it offers an alternative to conventional treatments that may involve medications with side effects or therapies that don't always work. For someone with a chronic autoimmune condition like PMR, the promise of herbal remedies can seem like a beacon of hope, especially when traditional treatments are limited, expensive, or simply not providing the desired relief.

Herbal remedies also carry the allure of being "natural." For patients who are skeptical of pharmaceuticals or weary from a long medical journey, the concept of healing through nature resonates deeply. The idea that the solution to their complex problems lies in simple, plant-based remedies is both comforting and empowering. However, while the appeal is understandable, it is crucial to recognize that "natural" does not always equate to "safe" or "effective."

Misleading Claims of Herbal Cures for PMR

The idea that herbal remedies can cure or significantly relieve symptoms of PMR is often touted by alternative health practitioners or through unregulated online platforms. These claims are typically not based on scientific research but rather on anecdotal evidence or outdated medical beliefs. Unfortunately, in the absence of a definitive cure for PMR, some patients may turn to these unverified treatments in a desperate attempt to manage their symptoms.

PMR is a condition marked by inflammation in the muscles and tissues around the shoulders and hips. It often causes pain and stiffness, particularly in the morning. Herbal remedies do not have the capacity to reverse this inflammatory process or alleviate the underlying cause of PMR. Any claims that herbs can reduce the inflammation, cure the condition, or replace corticosteroid therapy are scientifically unfounded and misleading. However, that hasn't stopped proponents from making these bold and irresponsible assertions.

Popular Herbs Promoted for PMR

Several herbs are commonly promoted as treatments for inflammatory conditions like PMR, even though there is no scientific evidence supporting their effectiveness. Below are some of the herbs frequently recommended by alternative practitioners for autoimmune or inflammatory issues:

1. **Turmeric (Curcumin):** Known for its anti-inflammatory properties, turmeric is often suggested as a treatment to reduce the inflammation associated with PMR. While turmeric may help reduce general inflammation, there is no evidence to suggest that it can replace corticosteroid

therapy or manage the systemic inflammation caused by PMR.

2. **Boswellia (Indian Frankincense):** Another anti-inflammatory herb, Boswellia is marketed as a remedy for reducing pain and swelling. Although it may have mild anti-inflammatory effects, it is not a substitute for the powerful medications required to manage PMR.

3. **Willow Bark:** Often promoted as a natural pain reliever due to its salicin content (a precursor to aspirin), willow bark may help with general aches and pains. However, it is not strong enough to address the significant pain and stiffness associated with PMR, and there are potential risks of bleeding for patients taking blood thinners.

4. **Ginger:** Ginger is widely known for its anti-inflammatory properties and is often recommended for arthritis-like conditions. While it may offer some relief for mild inflammation, it is not a treatment for the severe, systemic inflammation seen in PMR.

5. **Devil's Claw:** This herb is sometimes suggested for joint pain and inflammation. However, while it may provide mild relief for osteoarthritis, there is no clinical evidence to support its use in treating PMR.

The Danger of Interactions and Side Effects

One of the most pressing concerns about using herbal remedies to treat PMR is the potential for dangerous drug interactions and side effects. Patients with PMR are often prescribed corticosteroids, pain relievers, or other medications to manage their symptoms. Introducing herbal remedies into their regimen can interfere with these medications or lead to unexpected side effects.

For example:

- **St. John's Wort**, commonly used for depression, can interact with antidepressants, birth control pills, and blood thinners, reducing their efficacy.

- **Ginkgo Biloba**, as mentioned earlier, can increase bleeding risks, especially for patients taking anticoagulants.
- **Kava**, another herb used to alleviate anxiety, has been linked to serious liver damage and should not be used long-term or without medical supervision.

Moreover, the unregulated nature of herbal supplements poses additional risks. Unlike pharmaceutical medications, herbal supplements are not subjected to the same rigorous testing for safety, efficacy, or quality. This means that patients may be taking supplements that are mislabeled, contaminated, or contain inconsistent levels of active ingredients.

The Placebo Effect and Perceived Relief

One reason patients may feel temporary relief from herbal remedies is the placebo effect. The placebo effect occurs when a person experiences a perceived or actual improvement in their symptoms after receiving a treatment that has no therapeutic value. In the case of herbal remedies, patients might feel better simply because they believe the treatment is working, rather than because the herbs are providing any real relief.

For someone dealing with a chronic condition like PMR, which may cause intermittent symptoms such as pain and stiffness, the placebo effect can be particularly powerful. During periods of symptom fluctuation, patients might attribute a natural improvement to the herbal remedy, when in reality, the symptoms may have lessened on their own.

The Risks of Delaying Effective Treatment

One of the most dangerous aspects of relying on herbal remedies for PMR is the potential delay in receiving effective medical care. Herbal remedies may provide a false sense of security, leading patients to forgo or postpone treatments that could alleviate symptoms or prevent further damage.

PMR is typically treated with corticosteroids to reduce inflammation and pain. In some cases, additional medications are prescribed to manage symptoms or reduce the long-term effects of steroids. While corticosteroids can have side effects, they are often necessary to control the inflammation caused by PMR. Relying solely on herbal remedies, especially for a progressive condition, can lead to worsening symptoms, increased pain, and irreversible damage.

The Herbal Industry and Lack of Regulation

One reason herbal remedies are so widely available and marketed as cures for serious conditions like PMR is the lack of regulation in the supplement industry. In the United States, for example, the Food and Drug Administration (FDA) does not regulate herbal supplements in the same way it does prescription or over-the-counter medications. This lack of oversight means that manufacturers can make broad, unverified claims about the benefits of their products without being held to rigorous scientific standards.

As a result, patients may encounter websites, books, or alternative health practitioners who promote herbal remedies as a "cure" for PMR without any evidence to back up these claims. In some cases, these practitioners may genuinely believe in the power of herbs, while in others, they may be exploiting vulnerable patients for financial gain.

Herbal Medicine: When It Works, When It Doesn't

To be clear, not all herbal remedies are without value. Many pharmaceutical drugs are derived from plants, and some herbs do have scientifically documented benefits for certain conditions. For example, ginger is well-known for reducing nausea, and peppermint oil may help with irritable bowel syndrome. However, the key distinction is that these herbs have been studied in clinical trials and have specific, targeted uses.

The problem arises when herbal remedies are promoted as cures for conditions they cannot possibly address, such as PMR. A systemic inflammatory condition cannot be fixed with a plant-based remedy, no matter how potent the herb is. Herbal remedies may have a role in overall health, such as boosting the immune system or providing antioxidants, but they cannot reverse the inflammation caused by an autoimmune disorder.

Conclusion: Balancing Natural and Evidence-Based Medicine

Herbal remedies have their place in health and wellness, but they are not a cure-all, especially not for complex autoimmune conditions like PMR. Patients seeking relief must be cautious when navigating the world of alternative medicine, particularly when it comes to unverified claims and unregulated supplements. The best course of action is to combine the wisdom of natural health with evidence-based medicine, ensuring that your path to wellness is both safe and effective.

11 Uncredible Aromatherapy

The use of essential oils has surged in recent years, with proponents claiming that these fragrant extracts can alleviate a wide array of health problems. From headaches to anxiety, essential oils are marketed as natural, gentle solutions to a host of ailments. Their appeal is widespread, particularly for those seeking alternatives to traditional medicine. Among the many conditions that essential oils are claimed to treat is Polymyalgia Rheumatica (PMR), a chronic inflammatory disorder that affects muscles and joints. The idea that essential oils could provide relief for PMR symptoms such as pain, stiffness, and fatigue is alluring. However, these claims are not supported by credible scientific evidence.

In this chapter, we will explore the rise of essential oils as treatments, examine the pseudoscientific claims surrounding their use for PMR, and analyze the risks associated with relying on essential oils for serious medical conditions. While essential oils may have a place in certain aspects of wellness, their promotion as cures or treatments for conditions like PMR represents a dangerous form of quackery.

The Popularity of Essential Oils

Essential oils have been used for centuries in various cultures, primarily for their fragrance, cosmetic uses, and supposed therapeutic properties. In recent years, there has been a significant resurgence in their popularity, driven by the global wellness movement. Promoted by multi-level marketing companies and alternative health influencers, essential oils are now commonly found in homes, health food stores, and even mainstream retail outlets. The global essential oil market has grown exponentially, fueled by claims that these oils can relieve stress, boost immunity, improve sleep, and even treat chronic illnesses.

For people with chronic conditions like PMR, the appeal of a natural remedy is understandable. Living with daily pain, stiffness, and fatigue can be exhausting, and many patients seek out alternative treatments when conventional medicine doesn't provide the relief they hope for. Essential oils, with their soothing scents and association with relaxation, seem like a gentle, harmless option. But while they may help promote relaxation or reduce mild stress for some people, their use as a treatment for chronic inflammatory disorders like PMR is unfounded.

Claims of Essential Oils for PMR

The marketing of essential oils often makes bold claims, particularly when it comes to managing symptoms associated with PMR. The oils are often touted as able to alleviate pain, reduce inflammation, and ease stiffness—all common symptoms of PMR. Specific oils such as lavender, peppermint, eucalyptus, and frankincense are frequently promoted as powerful remedies that can address the discomfort associated with PMR.

For example, lavender oil is marketed as a natural remedy for stress and sleep disturbances, both of which can be secondary concerns for PMR patients. Peppermint oil is often suggested for muscle pain, with claims that applying it to the skin can reduce pain and stiffness. Frankincense is promoted for its supposed anti-inflammatory properties, with some suggesting that it can help with the inflammation in PMR. These oils are typically recommended for topical application, inhalation through diffusers, or even ingestion, with claims that they can penetrate the body's systems and provide relief at the source of the problem.

However, these claims are not backed by scientific evidence. While essential oils may have a place in certain wellness practices—such as aromatherapy for relaxation or mild stress relief—there is no credible research to support the idea that essential oils can alleviate the inflammation and pain associated with PMR.

The Pseudoscientific Foundation of Essential Oil Claims

The claims surrounding essential oils for PMR rest on a pseudoscientific foundation. Proponents of essential oils often cite their natural origins as proof of their safety and efficacy, conflating "natural" with "effective." This appeal to nature fallacy is common in alternative medicine, where the belief is that anything derived from nature must be beneficial to health.

The problem with this line of thinking is that it ignores the complexity of medical conditions like PMR. PMR is an inflammatory disorder where the immune system attacks healthy tissues, causing pain and stiffness. Essential oils, no matter how fragrant or soothing, cannot reverse this inflammatory process or alleviate the pain caused by PMR. Moreover, the idea that simply inhaling or applying an essential oil can treat such a complex condition lacks any scientific basis.

Research on essential oils has shown some mild benefits, particularly for reducing stress or anxiety, but this does not translate to treating chronic inflammatory conditions like PMR. The therapeutic use of essential oils for pain management, inflammation, or autoimmune disorders remains largely unproven. In the case of PMR, there is no scientific evidence to suggest that essential oils can alleviate the specific symptoms of the disorder.

Testimonials Versus Actual Outcomes

One of the reasons essential oils have gained such popularity is the abundance of testimonials from people who claim to have experienced significant benefits. These personal stories are powerful, often shared in online forums, social media groups, and through direct marketing efforts by essential oil companies. Testimonials from individuals who say that essential oils helped their pain or reduced their inflammation can be convincing, particularly for those who are desperate for relief.

However, it is important to distinguish between anecdotal evidence and scientific research. Testimonials, while compelling, do not provide reliable evidence of efficacy. They are often subject to the placebo effect, where a person believes they are feeling better simply because they expect the treatment to work. In the case of essential oils, the relaxing effect of inhaling a pleasant scent or the act of self-care in using a product may contribute to a perceived improvement in symptoms. This is not the same as a treatment that actually addresses the underlying medical condition.

Additionally, essential oil companies often rely on these personal stories to market their products, creating a feedback loop where more people try the oils based on anecdotal reports rather than evidence-based recommendations. This can be particularly dangerous for patients with serious medical conditions like PMR, who may be misled into thinking that essential oils can provide more than just a temporary placebo effect.

The Risks of Essential Oils for PMR Patients

While essential oils are generally considered safe when used properly, they are not without risks—particularly for individuals with serious medical conditions. Essential oils are highly concentrated plant extracts, and improper use can lead to adverse reactions. For PMR patients, the risks of relying on essential oils as a treatment can be significant.

First, essential oils cannot treat the underlying cause of PMR, which is systemic inflammation. By focusing on essential oils instead of pursuing evidence-based treatments, patients may delay or forgo the medical care they need. PMR often requires corticosteroids or other immunosuppressive medications to manage inflammation and prevent further damage. Delaying proper treatment can lead to worsening symptoms, including increased pain, stiffness, and reduced mobility.

Second, essential oils can cause allergic reactions or skin irritations, particularly when applied topically without proper dilution. Some oils, such as eucalyptus or peppermint, can cause respiratory issues if inhaled in large amounts or used around sensitive individuals. Ingesting essential oils, which is sometimes recommended by alternative practitioners, can be particularly dangerous, as these substances can be toxic in high concentrations.

Finally, the financial cost of essential oils can be a burden for patients, especially when they are marketed as ongoing treatments. Essential oils are often sold at high prices through multi-level marketing companies, which can put vulnerable patients in a position where they are spending significant amounts of money on products that provide no real benefit for their condition.

The Placebo Effect and Perceived Benefits

One of the reasons essential oils are so popular is the placebo effect, a well-documented phenomenon where patients experience perceived improvements in their condition simply because they believe a treatment will work. The placebo effect is not limited to essential oils—it occurs across all types of medicine, including pharmaceuticals. However, in the case of essential oils, the placebo effect is often mistaken for actual therapeutic benefit.

For PMR patients, the placebo effect can lead to a temporary reduction in anxiety, stress, or even perceived pain. This is particularly true when essential oils are used in conjunction with other relaxation techniques, such as meditation, massage, or a calming environment. However, this does not mean that essential oils are effectively treating the symptoms of PMR. The relief provided by the placebo effect is temporary and does not address the root cause of the condition.

The danger lies in mistaking the placebo effect for real improvement, which can prevent patients from seeking appropriate medical care. While relaxation and stress reduction are important aspects of managing chronic illness, they cannot replace medical treatments that are designed to address the physical and inflammatory aspects of PMR.

Conclusion: A False Sense of Security

Essential oils may offer temporary relaxation or stress relief, but they cannot treat the systemic inflammation and pain associated with PMR. The claims made by essential oil companies and alternative practitioners are not backed by scientific evidence, and relying on these products can delay necessary medical care. For PMR patients, it is important to approach any treatment with a critical eye and to rely on evidence-based medicine for managing symptoms and improving quality of life.

While essential oils may have a place in personal wellness practices, they should not be seen as a cure or even a reliable treatment for serious medical conditions. In the case of PMR, essential oils offer false hope at best and dangerous delays in care at worst. As with any medical treatment, patients should consult with qualified healthcare providers to ensure they are pursuing safe and effective therapies.

12 Needles and Nonsense

Acupuncture, an ancient practice rooted in traditional Chinese medicine, has become a popular alternative therapy for many modern ailments. From chronic pain to anxiety, proponents of acupuncture claim that this practice, which involves the insertion of thin needles into specific points on the body, can alleviate a wide array of conditions. In recent years, acupuncture has been promoted as a treatment for chronic inflammatory disorders, including Polymyalgia Rheumatica (PMR). Supporters of acupuncture argue that it can relieve symptoms such as muscle pain, stiffness, and fatigue—common issues for those with PMR. However, despite its long history and modern popularity, there is little scientific evidence to support acupuncture's efficacy for treating serious conditions like PMR.

This chapter will explore the origins of acupuncture, the claims made about its effectiveness for PMR, and the dangers of relying on acupuncture as a treatment. We will also examine the pseudoscientific foundation of acupuncture, the role of the placebo effect, and the risks associated with delaying proper medical care in favor of this alternative therapy.

The Origins and Practice of Acupuncture

Acupuncture has its roots in traditional Chinese medicine

(TCM), a system of healing that dates back thousands of years. According to TCM, the body has a vital life force called "qi" (pronounced "chee") that flows through pathways known as meridians. When the flow of qi is blocked or imbalanced, illness is believed to occur. Acupuncturists claim that by inserting needles into specific points along the meridians, they can restore the balance of qi, thereby promoting healing and alleviating symptoms.

In the modern world, acupuncture has evolved beyond its TCM origins. It is now widely practiced in Western countries, where it is often promoted as a treatment for pain management, stress relief, and various other conditions. In some cases, acupuncture is used as a complementary therapy alongside conventional treatments, but in other instances, it is promoted as a stand-alone solution for serious medical conditions.

Acupuncture's appeal lies in its non-invasive nature and the belief that it offers a "natural" form of healing. This aligns with the growing trend of patients seeking alternatives to pharmaceutical treatments or invasive medical procedures. However, while acupuncture may offer temporary relief for some symptoms, particularly pain, there is little evidence to support its use as a treatment for chronic inflammatory disorders like PMR.

Claims About Acupuncture for PMR

Proponents of acupuncture often claim that the practice can alleviate the symptoms associated with PMR, including muscle pain, stiffness, and fatigue. These symptoms are common among PMR patients, and managing them can be challenging, as traditional medications do not always provide sufficient relief. As a result, some PMR patients turn to acupuncture, hoping it will offer an alternative form of symptom management.

Acupuncturists argue that by stimulating certain points along the body's meridians, acupuncture can help "release" pain and reduce inflammation. Specific points on the shoulders, neck, and upper back are frequently targeted in treatments for PMR patients, as these are areas where pain and stiffness are often concentrated. Some acupuncturists even claim that acupuncture can improve circulation and reduce inflammation, which they argue could help alleviate the symptoms of PMR.

These claims, however, lack scientific backing. While some patients may experience temporary relief from acupuncture, there is no credible evidence to suggest that it can address the underlying inflammatory processes in PMR. Acupuncture cannot alter the fact that PMR is an autoimmune disorder, and the symptoms of pain and stiffness are caused by systemic inflammation, not blocked qi.

Acupuncture is based on concepts that have no grounding in modern scientific understanding of the human body. The notion of qi and meridians, for example, has never been demonstrated or observed in any scientific study. Despite centuries of practice, there is no anatomical or physiological evidence to support the idea that qi exists or that it flows through the body in specific channels.

Modern acupuncture has attempted to move away from its mystical roots by offering new explanations for how it works. Some acupuncturists claim that the insertion of needles stimulates the nervous system, releasing endorphins (the body's natural painkillers) or promoting blood flow to specific areas. However, these explanations are speculative at best. While the insertion of needles may cause a mild response from the nervous system—such as the release of endorphins—this effect is not specific to acupuncture points and does not explain how acupuncture would address the underlying inflammation caused by PMR.

Moreover, clinical trials on acupuncture have generally found that its effects are no better than placebo. In studies where participants received "sham" acupuncture—where needles are inserted randomly or superficially, without targeting traditional acupuncture points—patients reported similar levels of symptom relief as those who received real acupuncture. This suggests that the benefits of acupuncture are largely attributable to the placebo effect, rather than any specific therapeutic action.

The Placebo Effect and Acupuncture

The placebo effect is a well-documented phenomenon in which patients experience real improvements in their symptoms after receiving a treatment that has no therapeutic value. The power of the placebo effect lies in the patient's belief that the treatment will work. In the case of acupuncture, the ritual of the treatment—the careful placement of needles, the calm environment, and the practitioner's reassurance—can lead to a powerful placebo response.

For patients with PMR, the placebo effect can offer temporary relief from pain or discomfort. This is especially true for symptoms like muscle stiffness and fatigue, which are influenced by stress and anxiety. However, the placebo effect does not address the root cause of PMR, which is systemic inflammation.

The danger of relying on the placebo effect in the case of PMR is that it can give patients false hope. While they may feel better in the short term, their condition is not being treated, and their symptoms may worsen over time. The temporary relief provided by acupuncture can lead some patients to delay seeking appropriate medical care, which can have serious consequences for their long-term health.

Risks of Acupuncture for PMR Patients

While acupuncture is generally considered safe when performed by trained practitioners, it is not without risks—especially for patients with serious medical conditions like PMR. One of the main risks of acupuncture is the potential for infection. Because acupuncture involves inserting needles into the skin, there is always a risk of introducing bacteria into the body. This risk is heightened if the needles are not properly sterilized or if the practitioner does not follow proper hygiene protocols.

For PMR patients, who may already have compromised immune function due to steroid treatment, the risk of infection or other complications from acupuncture can be particularly concerning. In some cases, acupuncture has been associated with more serious adverse events, such as punctured organs or nerve damage, although these incidents are rare.

Another risk is that acupuncture may provide a false sense of security, leading patients to delay or avoid seeking evidence-based treatments. PMR is a condition that often requires corticosteroids or other medications to reduce inflammation and manage symptoms. Delaying appropriate medical care can result in worsening pain, increased stiffness, and reduced mobility.

Testimonials Versus Scientific Evidence

As with many alternative therapies, acupuncture is often promoted through personal testimonials rather than scientific evidence. Patients who report feeling better after acupuncture treatments may attribute their improvement to the needles, when in fact their symptoms may have improved on their own or as a result of the placebo effect. Testimonials can be persuasive, especially when they come from fellow patients who share similar struggles.

However, it is important to recognize the limitations of anecdotal evidence. Just because one person reports feeling better after acupuncture does not mean that the treatment is effective for everyone, or that it addresses the underlying cause of their condition. PMR is a complex inflammatory disorder that requires medical intervention, and there is no credible evidence to suggest that acupuncture can alter the course of the disease.

Moreover, the lack of regulation in the acupuncture industry means that patients may be vulnerable to unscrupulous practitioners who make exaggerated or false claims about the benefits of the treatment. Without proper oversight, it can be difficult for patients to distinguish between legitimate practitioners and those who are offering a service with no real therapeutic value.

One of the most concerning aspects of acupuncture for PMR is the false hope it offers to patients. PMR is a serious condition that can cause debilitating symptoms and, in some cases, long-term disability. Patients who are desperate for relief may turn to alternative therapies like acupuncture in the hopes of finding a cure or a treatment that will alleviate their suffering.

Unfortunately, acupuncture does not offer a cure for PMR. While it may provide temporary relief for some symptoms, it cannot address the systemic inflammation that is at the heart of the condition. Relying on acupuncture as a treatment can prevent patients from seeking the medical care they need, potentially leading to worse outcomes.

For patients with PMR, it is essential to pursue evidence-based treatments that have been proven to be effective in managing the condition. This may include medication, physical therapy, and, in some cases, lifestyle changes. While acupuncture may have a place in complementary care for managing stress or mild pain, it should not be viewed as a substitute for medical treatment.

Conclusion: Acupuncture and the Illusion of Healing

Acupuncture may offer a temporary reprieve from pain or discomfort, but it does not provide a solution for PMR. The practice is based on principles that lack scientific support, and its effects are largely attributable to the placebo effect. While acupuncture is generally safe, it carries risks for patients with serious medical conditions, and its promotion as a treatment for PMR represents a dangerous form of quackery.

For PMR patients, the most important step is to seek evidence-based treatments that address the underlying cause of their condition. While alternative therapies like acupuncture may offer short-term relief, they cannot replace the medical interventions that are necessary to manage the symptoms and progression of PMR. By focusing on proven treatments and working with qualified healthcare providers, patients can ensure that they are receiving the best possible care for their condition.

13 A Breath of False Hope

Ozone therapy has emerged as another alternative treatment that has been promoted for its supposed ability to cure a range of conditions, from chronic pain to infections and even serious autoimmune disorders. Proponents of ozone therapy claim that it can increase oxygen levels in the body, boost the immune system, and, in some cases, even reverse damage caused by inflammatory conditions such as Polymyalgia Rheumatica (PMR). However, like many alternative treatments, ozone therapy is not backed by credible scientific evidence, and in many cases, it can be dangerous. This chapter will explore the rise of ozone therapy, the claims made by its advocates, and the dangers it presents, especially for individuals with serious conditions like PMR.

The Origins and Concept of Ozone Therapy

Ozone (O_3) is a molecule composed of three oxygen atoms. While oxygen (O_2) is essential for life, ozone is a toxic gas when inhaled, as it is highly reactive and can cause significant damage to the respiratory tract. Despite its toxicity, ozone has been used for various industrial purposes, such as water purification and sterilization, due to its ability to kill bacteria and viruses. These industrial applications have led some alternative health practitioners to promote ozone as a potential therapy for medical conditions, under the false assumption that what kills bacteria and viruses in water or air might also heal the human body.

Ozone therapy involves introducing ozone into the body through various methods, including insufflation (blowing ozone into body cavities such as the rectum or vagina), injections, or autohemotherapy (where blood is drawn, mixed with ozone, and then re-injected into the patient). The goal of ozone therapy, according to its proponents, is to increase the amount of oxygen in the bloodstream, which they claim can help the body heal itself.

Advocates of ozone therapy argue that oxygen is vital for cellular function, and by introducing more oxygen into the body, it can fight off infections, reduce inflammation, and repair damaged tissues. Some practitioners even claim that ozone can "detoxify" the body, eliminating harmful substances and boosting overall health. These claims are enticing, especially for patients with chronic conditions like PMR, who may feel that conventional treatments are inadequate. However, ozone therapy is based on a flawed understanding of both medical science and the body's needs, and it carries significant risks.

Dubious Claims: Ozone Therapy for PMR

Ozone therapy is marketed as a potential treatment for a wide variety of conditions, including autoimmune diseases, chronic pain, and inflammatory disorders like PMR. For patients with PMR, the promises of ozone therapy can be particularly appealing. Practitioners claim that ozone therapy can reduce inflammation, relieve pain, and even improve immune function by increasing oxygen delivery to the affected tissues.

PMR is an autoimmune condition characterized by widespread muscle pain and stiffness, especially in the shoulders, neck, and hips. The cause is systemic inflammation, which is treated primarily with corticosteroids like prednisone to reduce inflammation and manage symptoms. Advocates of ozone therapy suggest that increasing oxygen levels in the bloodstream can enhance healing and reduce PMR symptoms by providing more oxygen to the muscles and joints.

Some ozone therapy practitioners claim that the treatment can reverse the effects of PMR by promoting the regeneration of damaged tissues and reducing inflammation. However, these claims are not supported by any credible scientific evidence. There is no plausible mechanism by which ozone therapy could alter the autoimmune processes associated with PMR, and the idea that increasing oxygen levels could somehow repair the damage caused by inflammation is simply not based in reality.

The Dangers of Ozone Therapy

Ozone therapy is not only ineffective for treating conditions like PMR; it is also potentially dangerous. Ozone is a toxic gas, and exposing the body to high concentrations of ozone can cause serious harm. Inhalation of ozone, even in small amounts, can irritate the respiratory system, leading to coughing, shortness of breath, and lung damage. When used internally through injections or insufflation, ozone can cause inflammation, tissue damage, and, in some cases, life-threatening complications.

One of the primary risks associated with ozone therapy is the potential for oxidative stress. Ozone is highly reactive, and when introduced into the body, it can lead to the production of free radicals—unstable molecules that can damage cells, proteins, and DNA. While the body has natural antioxidant systems to neutralize free radicals, overwhelming these systems with ozone can result in significant oxidative damage, contributing to inflammation and the breakdown of healthy tissues.

In patients with inflammatory conditions like PMR, the introduction of ozone into the body can be especially risky. PMR already involves systemic inflammation, and introducing ozone could exacerbate this inflammation, potentially worsening symptoms and increasing the risk of tissue damage.

In addition to oxidative stress, there is also the risk of

infection when ozone is introduced into the body through injections or autohemotherapy. Anytime the skin is pierced or blood is manipulated outside the body, there is a risk of introducing harmful bacteria or viruses into the bloodstream. This risk is heightened if the practitioner does not follow proper sterilization procedures, which is a concern in many alternative therapy settings.

Despite the bold claims made by proponents of ozone therapy, there is little to no scientific evidence to support its use for any medical condition, let alone for chronic inflammatory disorders like PMR. While ozone has been studied for its antimicrobial properties in certain industrial and environmental applications, these studies do not translate to medical treatments. There is no credible research demonstrating that ozone therapy can increase oxygen levels in the body in a meaningful way, nor is there any evidence that it can cure or alleviate the symptoms of PMR.

In fact, the U.S. Food and Drug Administration (FDA) has issued warnings against the use of ozone therapy, stating that ozone is a toxic gas with no known useful medical application. The FDA's stance is clear: "Ozone is a toxic gas with no known useful medical application in specific, adjunctive, or preventive therapy." Furthermore, the FDA has warned that the use of ozone in medical treatments can result in severe respiratory complications and other health problems.

The lack of peer-reviewed studies supporting ozone therapy is a major red flag. Most of the "evidence" cited by ozone therapy advocates comes from poorly designed studies, anecdotal reports, or non-scientific sources. In many cases, the studies that claim to support ozone therapy are conducted by individuals or organizations with a financial interest in promoting the treatment, leading to biased and unreliable results. Patients should be wary of any treatment that lacks rigorous scientific backing, especially when it is promoted as a cure for serious medical conditions like PMR.

The Role of the Placebo Effect

As with many alternative therapies, the placebo effect plays a significant role in the perceived benefits of ozone therapy. Patients who undergo ozone therapy may report feeling better after treatment, but this improvement is often due to the placebo effect rather than any actual physiological changes. The placebo effect occurs when a patient's belief in the effectiveness of a treatment leads to real improvements in symptoms, even if the treatment itself has no therapeutic value.

For patients with chronic conditions like PMR, the placebo effect can be particularly powerful. Living with constant pain, fatigue, and stiffness can be exhausting, and the promise of a new treatment that offers hope can be enough to make patients feel better, at least temporarily. However, while the placebo effect can provide short-term relief, it does not address the underlying cause of the condition. Patients who rely on ozone therapy may feel better for a time, but their symptoms are likely to return, and the progression of their condition will continue unchecked.

The Ethical Implications of Ozone Therapy

One of the most troubling aspects of ozone therapy is the ethical implications of promoting a treatment that has no scientific backing and carries significant risks. Patients with PMR are often desperate for relief, especially if conventional treatments have failed to provide adequate symptom management. This desperation can make them vulnerable to unscrupulous practitioners who offer false hope in the form of unproven therapies like ozone.

By promoting ozone therapy as a cure for PMR, practitioners are taking advantage of patients' desperation and willingness to try anything that might offer relief. In many cases, these practitioners charge high fees for ozone treatments, despite the lack of evidence supporting their efficacy. This not only wastes patients' money but also diverts them from pursuing legitimate medical treatments that could actually improve their condition.

The ethical concerns surrounding ozone therapy extend

beyond financial exploitation. Patients who undergo ozone therapy may delay or forgo conventional treatments, believing that ozone will cure their condition. This can lead to worsening symptoms and preventable complications, especially in patients with progressive conditions like PMR. The promotion of unproven therapies like ozone is not only unethical but also dangerous, as it can cause real harm to patients who are already struggling with serious health issues.

Conclusion: Ozone Therapy as a False Hope

Ozone therapy is yet another alternative treatment that offers false hope to patients with serious medical conditions like PMR. Despite its claims of increasing oxygen levels, reducing inflammation, and promoting healing, there is no credible scientific evidence to support the use of ozone therapy for any medical condition. In fact, ozone therapy carries significant risks, including oxidative stress, infection, and respiratory complications.

For patients with PMR, the promises of ozone therapy are particularly dangerous. PMR is a chronic inflammatory condition that requires careful medical management, and relying on unproven therapies like ozone can delay or prevent patients from receiving the treatments they need. While the placebo effect may offer temporary relief, it does not address the underlying cause of the condition, and patients who pursue ozone therapy may ultimately be putting their health at risk.

As with any medical treatment, it is important for patients to critically evaluate the evidence behind ozone therapy and other alternative treatments. By seeking out scientifically validated treatments and working with qualified healthcare providers, patients can ensure that they are receiving the best possible care for their condition, rather than falling prey to false hope and pseudoscience.

14 How to Research on Your Own

When diagnosed with a complex condition like Polymyalgia Rheumatica (PMR), finding accurate and reliable information becomes crucial for navigating treatment options and making informed decisions about your health. The internet is saturated with a mix of credible scientific resources and misleading pseudoscience. For patients with PMR, knowing how to research properly and avoid misinformation can make a significant difference in your treatment and quality of life.

This chapter will provide you with essential tools to critically evaluate medical information on PMR, navigate peer-reviewed journals, and understand statistics so that you can discern which studies are credible. We will also explore how to avoid "quack" journals and pseudoscientific articles disguised as legitimate sources of medical research.

Understanding Peer-Reviewed Journals

The term "peer-reviewed" is often held as the gold standard for scientific literature. A peer-reviewed journal means that before a study is published, it is reviewed by other experts in the same field (peers) to assess its methodology, accuracy, and contribution to the existing body of research. However, not all journals that claim to be peer-reviewed are reputable, and not all peer-reviewed studies are flawless.

Characteristics of a Legitimate Peer-Reviewed Journal

- **Reputation**: Real peer-reviewed journals are usually affiliated with reputable academic institutions, organizations, or well-established publishers such as Wiley, Springer, Elsevier, or the Nature Publishing Group. You can typically recognize legitimate journals by checking if their publisher is well-known and respected.

- **Impact Factor**: The impact factor of a journal measures how often articles published in that journal are cited by other researchers. While not a perfect metric, journals with a higher impact factor tend to be more reputable. A journal with an impact factor above 1.0 is generally considered credible, while prestigious medical journals like *The Lancet* or *New England Journal of Medicine* may have impact factors above 50.

- **Indexed in Databases**: Legitimate peer-reviewed journals are indexed in reputable databases such as PubMed, Scopus, and Web of Science. These databases have stringent criteria for listing journals, making it unlikely that predatory or pseudoscientific journals will appear in their databases.

How to Spot Predatory or Quack Journals

Unfortunately, the rise of the internet has made it easier for pseudo-journals, or "predatory journals," to masquerade as legitimate sources of scientific information. These journals may claim to be peer-reviewed, but they often lack scientific integrity and are driven by financial motives.

Red Flags of Predatory Journals:

- **Unsolicited Emails**: If you receive emails inviting you to submit papers or review articles for a journal you've never heard of, this is often a sign of a predatory journal. Legitimate journals do not typically solicit papers in this manner.

- **High Fees**: Predatory journals often charge exorbitant

publication fees, sometimes up to several thousand dollars. While some reputable journals charge fees, especially open-access ones, predatory journals exist primarily to collect these fees and may skip the peer-review process entirely.

- **Quick Review Process**: If a journal claims that your submission will be reviewed and published within just a few days or a week, this is a red flag. Proper peer review takes time, often months, to carefully assess the study's methodology and findings.

- **Lack of Transparency**: Predatory journals often lack transparency about their peer-review process, editorial board members, and affiliations. If you cannot easily find information about the editorial board or the journal's affiliations, it's best to steer clear.

- **Flawed or Non-Existent Review Process**: These journals may publish articles without genuine peer review, leading to misleading, unsupported, or even dangerous conclusions.

Navigating Statistics and Medical Research

Reading a medical journal article is one thing; understanding it is another. Many journal articles include complex statistics that can be difficult to interpret. Learning how to understand basic statistics can help you determine whether the findings are meaningful or misleading.

Key Statistical Terms to Know

- **P-Value**: The p-value is a measure of the probability that the results of a study are due to chance. A p-value of less than 0.05 is often considered statistically significant, but statistical significance does not always equate to clinical significance.

- **Confidence Interval (CI)**: A confidence interval provides a range of values within which the true result likely falls. A narrow CI suggests more precise results, while a wide CI indicates less certainty.

- **Sample Size**: The number of participants in a study matters. Larger sample sizes provide more reliable results, while small samples may not be generalizable and can produce misleading conclusions.
- **Relative Risk (RR) and Odds Ratio (OR)**: These measure the strength of an association between a treatment and an outcome. A relative risk of 1.0 means no difference, while values greater than 1.0 suggest increased risk and values less than 1.0 suggest decreased risk.

Identifying Reliable Research

Once you understand the basics, you can critically evaluate individual research articles. Look for these indicators:

- **Randomized Controlled Trials (RCTs)**: These are the gold standard for clinical research. In these studies, participants are randomly assigned to either the treatment or control group, reducing bias.
- **Meta-Analyses and Systematic Reviews**: These compile data from multiple studies to draw broader conclusions. They are considered more reliable because they provide a comprehensive view of existing research.
- **Peer Review by Experts in the Field**: Check the author credentials. Are they respected researchers in PMR or related fields? If the study is peer-reviewed by experts, it is more likely to be trustworthy.
- **Funding Source**: Be cautious of studies funded by organizations with a financial interest in the outcome. Potential conflicts of interest should be disclosed in the study.

How to Spot Misleading Research and False Statistics

Some studies are designed to manipulate statistics or selectively report data. Watch out for:

- **Cherry-Picking Data**: Reporting only favorable results while ignoring others can create the illusion that a treatment is more effective than it is.

- **Too Good to Be True**: Studies that report miraculous cures should be treated with caution.
- **Lack of Control Group**: Without a control group, it's impossible to know if the treatment is effective.
- **Small Sample Size or Short Duration**: Studies with few participants or short follow-up periods may not provide reliable results.
- **Conflicts of Interest**: Always check if the study was funded by a company that stands to profit from positive results.

Using Quackwatch and Other Resources to Avoid Pseudoscience

To avoid falling prey to pseudoscientific treatments, use trusted resources like Quackwatch, a nonprofit organization dedicated to exposing pseudoscientific health claims. Quackwatch provides information on a wide range of alternative therapies, highlighting the lack of evidence behind many popular treatments.

Other reliable resources include:

- **National Institutes of Health (NIH)**: Provides extensive resources on health topics, including PMR.
- **Cochrane Library**: Publishes systematic reviews of clinical trials, offering high-quality evidence on treatments.
- **PubMed**: A database of biomedical literature, including reputable peer-reviewed journals.

Conclusion

Navigating medical research can be overwhelming, especially with a complex condition like PMR. By understanding peer-reviewed journals, basic statistics, and how to spot pseudoscience, you can make more informed decisions. Always critically evaluate the sources and consult reliable resources like Quackwatch and PubMed to ensure that you are making decisions based on sound science rather than pseudoscience. By doing so, you can avoid falling prey to false hope and quackery, ensuring the best care for your condition.

15 Proven Treatments for PMR

Polymyalgia Rheumatica (PMR) is a chronic inflammatory condition that primarily affects the muscles, leading to pain, stiffness, and discomfort, especially in the shoulders, neck, and hips. While there is no cure for PMR, various treatments can help manage symptoms, improve quality of life, and prevent complications. According to the Mayo Clinic, effective management often involves a combination of medication, lifestyle changes, and regular monitoring. This chapter will outline 15 proven treatments for PMR, focusing on both medication-based and supportive therapies to help patients navigate their treatment journey and avoid unproven remedies.

1. Corticosteroids

Corticosteroids, particularly prednisone, are the first line of treatment for PMR. These medications help reduce inflammation and alleviate pain and stiffness in the muscles. Prednisone is typically prescribed at a low dose and gradually tapered off as symptoms improve. Most patients experience significant relief within days of starting treatment.

However, long-term use of corticosteroids can have side

effects, such as weight gain, high blood pressure, and increased risk of infections. Doctors must balance these risks with the benefits, and regular monitoring is essential to ensure the lowest effective dose is used.

2. Methotrexate

For patients who are unable to taper off corticosteroids or those who experience significant side effects, methotrexate may be prescribed as a corticosteroid-sparing agent. Methotrexate is an immunosuppressant that helps reduce inflammation and allows for lower doses of steroids.

While methotrexate is generally well-tolerated, it can cause side effects such as nausea, fatigue, and liver toxicity. Regular blood tests are required to monitor liver function and ensure the drug is being tolerated safely.

3. Nonsteroidal Anti-Inflammatory Drugs (NSAIDs)

While corticosteroids are the primary treatment for PMR, NSAIDs like ibuprofen and naproxen can be used to manage mild pain and inflammation. NSAIDs are not a substitute for corticosteroids in treating PMR but can be helpful for patients experiencing minor discomfort or as a supplementary treatment.

Long-term use of NSAIDs carries risks, including stomach ulcers, kidney damage, and increased cardiovascular risk. Patients should use NSAIDs only as directed by their doctor and avoid overuse.

4. Physical Therapy

Physical therapy is an important aspect of managing PMR, particularly for maintaining mobility and preventing muscle stiffness. A physical therapist can develop a personalized exercise program to improve flexibility, strength, and range of motion. Gentle stretching exercises can help alleviate stiffness, while low-impact aerobic activities, such as walking or swimming, can improve overall fitness.

Physical therapy can also reduce the risk of long-term complications, such as muscle weakness or joint immobility, which are common in patients with PMR due to prolonged inactivity.

5. Lifestyle Modifications

Lifestyle modifications play a critical role in managing PMR. Patients should prioritize regular, low-impact exercise to maintain muscle strength and joint flexibility. Avoiding activities that strain the muscles or joints, such as heavy lifting or repetitive motions, can help prevent exacerbation of symptoms.

Patients should also adopt a balanced diet rich in anti-inflammatory foods, including fruits, vegetables, lean proteins, and omega-3 fatty acids. Maintaining a healthy weight is important for reducing pressure on joints and muscles, especially in older adults.

6. Calcium and Vitamin D Supplements

Corticosteroid use can lead to decreased bone density, increasing the risk of osteoporosis in PMR patients. To mitigate this risk, doctors often recommend calcium and vitamin D supplements. These supplements help support bone health and reduce the likelihood of fractures.

Regular bone density scans may be required to monitor bone health, particularly for patients on long-term corticosteroid therapy.

7. Bisphosphonates

In addition to calcium and vitamin D supplements, bisphosphonates may be prescribed to protect against bone loss in patients taking corticosteroids for extended periods. Bisphosphonates, such as alendronate, help strengthen bones and reduce the risk of osteoporosis-related fractures.

As with any medication, bisphosphonates can have side effects, including gastrointestinal issues and rare complications such as osteonecrosis of the jaw. Regular dental check-ups are advised for patients taking these medications.

8. Regular Monitoring and Blood Tests

Patients with PMR need regular follow-up appointments to monitor their response to treatment and adjust medication dosages as necessary. Blood tests, including erythrocyte sedimentation rate (ESR) and C-reactive protein (CRP), are commonly used to measure inflammation levels in the body.

In addition to monitoring inflammation, doctors may check for side effects related to corticosteroid use, such as elevated blood sugar, cholesterol levels, or liver function abnormalities.

9. Occupational Therapy

PMR can make everyday tasks challenging due to muscle pain and stiffness. Occupational therapy helps patients adapt to these limitations by teaching them techniques to conserve energy and modify tasks to reduce strain on the muscles and joints.

Occupational therapists can recommend assistive devices, such as ergonomic tools or reachers, to help patients with activities like dressing, cooking, or cleaning, allowing them to maintain independence.

10. Cognitive Behavioral Therapy (CBT)

Living with a chronic condition like PMR can lead to emotional distress, including anxiety and depression. Cognitive Behavioral Therapy (CBT) is a proven psychological treatment that helps patients manage the emotional effects of chronic pain and fatigue.

CBT focuses on changing negative thought patterns and behaviors, helping patients develop coping strategies for the mental health challenges associated with PMR. By improving mental resilience, patients can better manage their condition and improve their overall well-being.

11. Hydrotherapy

Hydrotherapy, or water-based therapy, can be particularly beneficial for PMR patients who experience joint stiffness and muscle pain. The buoyancy of water reduces the strain on joints, allowing for gentle exercise that improves flexibility and strength without causing additional discomfort.

Many patients find that warm water therapy, such as in a heated pool, provides relief from muscle stiffness and improves their range of motion.

12. Massage Therapy

Massage therapy can offer temporary relief from muscle tension and pain in PMR patients. Gentle massage techniques help improve blood flow, reduce muscle stiffness, and promote relaxation. While massage therapy is not a cure for PMR, it can be a helpful complementary treatment for managing discomfort.

It's important for patients to consult with their healthcare provider before starting massage therapy to ensure it is appropriate for their condition.

13. Stress Management Techniques

Chronic pain and fatigue can be exacerbated by stress, making it important for PMR patients to develop stress management techniques. Practices such as mindfulness meditation, deep breathing exercises, or yoga can help patients manage stress and improve their overall quality of life.

These techniques not only reduce stress but can also help patients manage the emotional and physical symptoms of PMR more effectively.

14. Patient Education and Support Groups

Patient education is crucial for managing PMR. Understanding the condition, treatment options, and potential side effects of medications can help patients take an active role in their care. Doctors and healthcare teams should provide comprehensive information about the disease and how to manage it effectively.

Support groups also provide emotional support and practical advice from others living with PMR. Whether online or in-person, these groups can help patients connect with others facing similar challenges and share strategies for coping with the condition.

15. Pain Management Clinics

For patients with severe or persistent pain that is not well-managed with standard medications, pain management clinics offer specialized care. These clinics use a multidisciplinary approach to pain management, including medications, physical therapy, psychological support, and interventional treatments such as nerve blocks or injections.

Patients referred to a pain management clinic can benefit from tailored treatment plans that address both the physical and emotional aspects of chronic pain.

Avoiding Quackery and Misinformation

While these 15 treatments are proven to be effective for managing PMR, it's essential to avoid unproven or dangerous alternatives that promise cures or miracle treatments. As previously discussed, quack therapies often offer false hope and can lead patients away from necessary medical interventions.

By focusing on evidence-based treatments and working closely with their healthcare team, patients can manage their symptoms, improve their quality of life, and steer clear of the false promises of PMR quackery.

17 FAQ

Polymyalgia Rheumatica Quackery: Frequently Asked Questions

1. What is Polymyalgia Rheumatica (PMR), and how does it affect the body?

Polymyalgia Rheumatica (PMR) is a chronic inflammatory disorder that causes muscle pain and stiffness, especially in the shoulders, neck, and hips. It primarily affects people over the age of 50 and often involves significant morning stiffness. While the exact cause of PMR is unknown, it is considered an autoimmune condition, where the immune system mistakenly targets the body's own tissues. PMR symptoms can fluctuate, and without treatment, the condition can severely impact daily life and mobility.

2. What are the standard treatments for PMR?

The mainstay of PMR treatment is corticosteroids, such as prednisone, which help reduce inflammation and relieve pain. Most patients experience improvement within days of starting treatment, though corticosteroids may be needed for extended periods. Some patients may also take methotrexate or other immunosuppressants to reduce the steroid dose needed over time. In addition to medication, physical therapy and lifestyle adjustments, like low-impact exercise, may be recommended to help manage symptoms.

3. Can PMR be cured with diet alone?

No. While dietary adjustments, like anti-inflammatory foods, can help support overall health, no diet can cure PMR. PMR is an autoimmune disease, and dietary changes alone are not sufficient to control the inflammation. However, a balanced diet that reduces processed foods and emphasizes whole foods may help manage symptoms. Always consult your doctor or a registered dietitian before making any significant dietary changes, especially if they involve restrictive diets.

4. What are some warning signs of quack treatments for PMR?

Quack treatments often use vague, scientific-sounding language and make promises of quick cures. Warning signs include:

- Claims to "cure" PMR, a chronic condition that can only be managed, not cured.
- Reliance on testimonials instead of scientific research.
- Use of terms like "detox," "natural cure," or "holistic realignment."
- Expensive supplements or treatments with no clinical backing. If a treatment sounds too good to be true, it likely is.

5. Is Craniosacral Therapy (CST) a legitimate treatment for PMR?

No, Craniosacral Therapy is not a scientifically validated treatment for PMR. CST is based on the pseudoscientific idea that manipulating the bones in the skull can correct "craniosacral rhythms." This concept has no basis in anatomy or physiology, as the cranial bones are fused and cannot be manipulated to affect chronic conditions like PMR. Relying on CST instead of proven medical treatments could delay proper care and worsen symptoms.

6. Why are patients with PMR drawn to alternative treatments?

The chronic nature of PMR, combined with the side effects of long-term steroid use, can lead patients to seek alternative treatments. Additionally, PMR's fluctuating symptoms and periods of pain relief followed by flare-ups may cause frustration, prompting patients to look for solutions outside of conventional medicine. Quack practitioners often exploit this by offering false hope or "miracle cures."

7. Is it safe to stop my corticosteroids if I want to try an alternative treatment?

Stopping corticosteroids abruptly can be dangerous and may lead to severe flare-ups or withdrawal symptoms. Always consult your doctor before making any changes to your medication regimen. Abruptly discontinuing corticosteroids can cause a rapid worsening of symptoms, increased inflammation, and can even lead to serious complications.

8. Are there any safe complementary treatments for PMR?

Complementary treatments, when used alongside conventional medicine, may provide additional support. Low-impact exercise, physical therapy, and stress management techniques, like yoga and meditation, can be beneficial in managing PMR symptoms. Discuss any complementary treatments with your healthcare provider to ensure they are safe and will not interfere with your medication.

9. Can supplements help with PMR symptoms?

While certain supplements, like omega-3 fatty acids and turmeric, have mild anti-inflammatory properties, they are not replacements for prescribed medications. Supplements can interact with medications, so it's important to discuss any supplement use with your doctor. Avoid any supplement that claims to cure PMR or promises dramatic results, as these claims are usually unsubstantiated.

10. How can I verify if a treatment is legitimate?

Use credible medical sources like PubMed, the National Institutes of Health (NIH), and reputable organizations like the Mayo Clinic to research treatments. Systematic reviews and studies published in peer-reviewed journals are the gold standard for evaluating a treatment's legitimacy. Additionally, discussing potential therapies with your healthcare provider can help confirm whether they are evidence-based.

11. Are there any specific diets recommended for PMR patients?

While no specific diet will cure PMR, an anti-inflammatory diet may support general health and reduce some inflammation. This includes eating foods rich in omega-3s (such as fatty fish), antioxidants (found in fruits and vegetables), and avoiding processed foods, refined sugars, and trans fats. Patients should consult a nutritionist or dietitian before starting any restrictive diet.

12. What role does stress play in PMR symptoms?

Stress does not cause PMR, but it can exacerbate symptoms by increasing inflammation. High-stress levels can negatively affect immune function and may lead to flare-ups. Techniques like mindfulness, yoga, or deep breathing exercises may help reduce stress and, in turn, could alleviate some PMR symptoms.

13. Can acupuncture help with PMR?

Acupuncture is sometimes used as a complementary treatment for chronic pain. While some patients report temporary pain relief, acupuncture does not address the underlying inflammation of PMR. Evidence supporting its effectiveness is limited, and it should not be used as a replacement for proven medical treatments.

14. Why do some patients feel better after trying alternative treatments?

The placebo effect can make people feel temporarily better, as the belief in a treatment's effectiveness can create a psychological boost. Additionally, PMR symptoms can fluctuate naturally, so periods of improvement may coincide with trying a new alternative therapy. However, these improvements are usually short-lived if the treatment lacks a scientific basis.

15. Should I avoid all alternative treatments?

Not necessarily. Complementary treatments can be beneficial if they are used to support your overall wellness and do not interfere with proven medical treatments. For example, gentle exercise, massage, or mindfulness can support your mental and physical health. However, avoid any alternative treatments that claim to cure PMR or replace prescribed medication.

16. How can I tell if a website or health provider is trustworthy?

Trustworthy health providers and websites:

- Are associated with reputable institutions or medical organizations.

- Provide clear references to peer-reviewed research.

- Use straightforward language without sensationalist claims. Avoid sites that rely heavily on testimonials, promise quick cures, or sell expensive products as part of their "treatment."

17. Is it okay to take herbs or herbal supplements for PMR?

Some herbs, like turmeric, have mild anti-inflammatory properties but are not substitutes for medication. Herbal supplements can interact with prescribed medications, so it's essential to consult your healthcare provider before adding any new supplements to your regimen. Avoid herbs or supplements that promise to cure PMR or significantly reduce inflammation without scientific backing.

18. What are the risks of detox diets for PMR?

Detox diets, often promoted as ways to "cleanse" the body, lack scientific support and can be harmful. They may involve fasting or extreme dietary restrictions that can lead to malnutrition, dehydration, and electrolyte imbalances. For PMR patients, detox diets offer no benefit and can lead to more harm than good.

19. Why are testimonials so convincing, and should I trust them?

Testimonials are compelling because they feature real people sharing personal stories. However, they are often biased, selective, and not representative of scientific evidence. Personal experiences cannot replace clinical research, which considers a treatment's effect across large, diverse groups. Be cautious about testimonials promoting cures for PMR, especially when accompanied by unverified claims.

20. How can I make sure I am choosing the best treatment plan for my PMR?

The best treatment plan for PMR is one that is evidence-based, created with the guidance of healthcare professionals, and tailored to your unique needs. Stay informed, seek out reputable sources, ask your doctor questions, and be cautious about treatments not supported by scientific research. Taking an active role in your healthcare can help you avoid quack treatments and find the most effective strategies for managing your PMR.

17 Conclusion

As we conclude our exploration of Polymyalgia Rheumatica (PMR) and the challenges of navigating treatment options, it's essential to be well-equipped to identify pseudoscientific claims that promise "miracle cures." For patients managing PMR, the allure of quick fixes can be tempting, especially given the ongoing nature of this inflammatory condition and the side effects of conventional treatments. However, being able to distinguish credible, evidence-based medicine from unsupported claims not only safeguards your health but empowers you to make decisions rooted in scientific integrity.

Understanding the Risks of Pseudoscience for PMR Patients

Living with a serious medical condition like PMR presents significant challenges that extend beyond physical symptoms. The unpredictability of flare-ups, side effects of medications, and limited options for curative treatment can lead patients to search for alternative solutions. Unfortunately, these uncertainties create fertile ground for pseudoscientific treatments. In a landscape where misinformation can be easily accessed online, it's important to recognize the signs of pseudoscience and be cautious about treatments that lack scientific validation.

The Importance of Evidence-Based Medicine

Evidence-based medicine (EBM) forms the cornerstone of legitimate healthcare. It is grounded in rigorous scientific research, peer-reviewed studies, and clinical trials that confirm both efficacy and safety. The process of validating medical treatments is exhaustive, ensuring that they are not only effective but safe for patients. Treatments must withstand scrutiny through controlled studies and replication of results across multiple trials before they can be recommended as standard practice.

In contrast, pseudoscientific therapies lack scientific credibility. These "treatments" often rely on anecdotal claims, unverified testimonials, and pseudoscientific jargon to attract patients. Unfortunately, pseudoscience may sometimes exploit patients' trust, offering unsupported claims of "cures" that can mislead those in search of real solutions. This chapter aims to help you critically evaluate such claims and to confidently choose treatments that align with credible scientific evidence.

Recognizing Warning Signs of Pseudoscientific Treatments

To help you distinguish between valid treatments and pseudoscientific claims, here are several prominent red flags to consider:

- **Overly Optimistic Results:** Be wary of treatments that guarantee a cure for PMR or claim rapid, miraculous improvements. PMR is a complex autoimmune disease that can be managed but not cured outright.
- **Lack of Peer-Reviewed Research:** If you can't find any studies on the proposed treatment in reputable medical journals or databases, be suspicious. Credible treatments are documented and available for public scrutiny.
- **Equivocal Language:** Terms like "energy healing," "detoxifying the body," or "holistic re-alignment" often indicate a lack of scientific backing.
- **Reliance on Personal Testimonials:** Testimonials can be highly persuasive but are often cherry-picked and biased,

lacking the rigorous testing required to verify their validity. These are not a substitute for scientific evidence.

Steps to Evaluate a Potential Therapy

Whether you encounter a new treatment online, in conversation, or even in a book, taking a few essential steps can help you determine its legitimacy:

1. **Check Reputable Medical Databases**
   Resources like PubMed, a database maintained by the National Institutes of Health (NIH), host millions of peer-reviewed studies. If a treatment has credible support, it is likely to be documented in such databases. To check, visit PubMed.gov and search using terms like "Polymyalgia Rheumatica treatment." Any valid findings will likely be published here.

2. **Consult Reputable Health Organizations**
   Trusted health organizations such as the Mayo Clinic, National Institutes of Health, and the Centers for Disease Control and Prevention (CDC) maintain up-to-date information on proven treatments. They also evaluate the safety of alternative treatments, providing a reliable starting point for evaluating options. Many of these organizations offer resources that can clarify what is and isn't effective for PMR.

3. **Talk to Your Healthcare Provider**
   It's always wise to discuss new treatments with a qualified healthcare provider, particularly one familiar with your specific needs. Most physicians can provide insight into why certain treatments may not be suitable or potentially harmful for PMR patients. Consider asking questions like:
   - *What evidence is there to support this treatment?*
   - *Is there any known risk associated with it?*
   - *Do you believe this approach aligns with my overall treatment plan?*

4. **Look for Systematic Reviews and Consensus**

Statements

Systematic reviews evaluate large amounts of research to judge the effectiveness of treatments. For example, The Cochrane Library conducts reviews on health interventions and provides in-depth evaluations of different treatments. For PMR, searching for consensus statements or systematic reviews from reputable sources can reveal whether a proposed therapy holds any real merit.

5. **Avoid "Miracle Cure" Books and Articles**
   Books and articles that promise to "cure" PMR through extreme diets or unproven treatments should be viewed with skepticism. While dietary adjustments may contribute to improved quality of life, they are not a cure for autoimmune conditions like PMR. These materials often promote false hope, and their claims are usually unsupported by any scientific evidence.

Red Flags in Language and Marketing

Pseudoscientific claims often use language designed to appeal to the emotions of patients. Marketing terms like "revolutionary breakthrough," "all-natural cure," and "ancient healing secrets" are intended to evoke a sense of exclusivity and mystery. However, legitimate treatments do not rely on such language. Instead, they are communicated through straightforward, clinical explanations and backed by transparent data. When evaluating potential treatments, look for clear, specific descriptions of how the therapy works. A vague or "too good to be true" description is often an indicator of pseudoscience.

Protecting Your Health and Your Wallet

Many pseudoscientific treatments, especially those marketed online, come with a high price tag. For example, specialized "detox" programs or elaborate diet plans may promise benefits but require ongoing, costly purchases. For patients already managing healthcare expenses, these costs can quickly accumulate without yielding real benefits. Investing in unproven treatments not only risks your health but can also drain financial resources that would be better spent on proven therapies.

Trusting Science, Not Trends

The allure of alternative treatments for chronic illnesses is understandable. Chronic pain, fatigue, and the frustration of ongoing symptoms can drive patients to seek solutions beyond conventional medicine. Unfortunately, many of these "solutions" are built on popular health trends rather than hard science. By understanding the basis of evidence-based medicine and applying critical thinking to new treatment options, you can avoid falling victim to fleeting trends or false promises.

Be Wary of Anecdotal Evidence

Anecdotal evidence is one of the most commonly used tactics in pseudoscientific marketing. Stories of "miraculous recoveries" or "life-changing results" can be emotionally compelling, but they lack the rigorous testing and statistical analysis required to determine a treatment's true effectiveness. For PMR patients, personal testimonials are no replacement for the research conducted through clinical trials. While it's tempting to trust firsthand experiences, anecdotal evidence is too subjective and too prone to bias to be considered reliable.

The Role of Patient Support Communities

For patients dealing with chronic conditions like PMR, finding support through online communities can be valuable. However, these forums can also be breeding grounds for misinformation. When participating in online discussions, it's essential to critically assess any medical advice offered and remember that other patients' experiences may not reflect scientifically validated outcomes. Support groups can provide emotional support but should not be a substitute for professional medical guidance.

Final Thoughts: Navigating the Landscape of PMR Treatments

As we close this chapter, remember that while the treatment journey for PMR is challenging, adhering to evidence-based medicine is the best course of action. It's easy to feel overwhelmed by the conflicting information and promises of quick fixes that pervade alternative medicine. However, by grounding your choices in credible research and professional guidance, you're safeguarding not only your health but also your sense of agency in managing PMR.

Living with PMR involves balancing medical treatments, lifestyle adjustments, and sometimes, difficult trade-offs. While no treatment currently offers a cure, the path to managing PMR lies in adhering to methods proven through clinical research. Avoiding pseudoscience and understanding the limitations and strengths of various therapies will help you take a well-informed and empowered approach to your health. With vigilance, knowledge, and support from qualified healthcare providers, you can navigate the challenges of PMR without falling prey to false promises.

Key Takeaways for PMR Patients:

- **Trust Science:** Prioritize treatments backed by clinical research and peer-reviewed studies.

- **Stay Informed:** Regularly consult credible sources like the NIH, Mayo Clinic, and PubMed.

- **Avoid "Miracle Cures":** Be cautious of any treatment that promises quick or guaranteed results.

- **Consult Healthcare Providers:** Engage in open discussions with your doctor before trying new therapies.

- **Maintain Critical Thinking:** Be skeptical of anecdotal evidence, testimonials, and persuasive marketing.

By adhering to these principles, you ensure that your journey toward better health is both safe and grounded in evidence, helping you manage PMR effectively and avoid the pitfalls of pseudoscience.

About the Authors

Cheryl White has been a dedicated health science writer for more than 30 years. With an undergraduate degree in Health Sciences and two master's degrees, Cheryl's passion for helping people live healthier lives comes through in her writing, making complex health issues understandable and accessible for all readers.

Shane Wilson is a dedicated medical professional with a passion for debunking health myths and pseudoscientific practices. With over three years of experience in crafting well-researched, engaging medical content, Shane aims to empower readers with accurate, evidence-based information. His writing is a compelling blend of expertise and clarity, making complex medical topics accessible to all.

Printed in Great Britain
by Amazon